The UK's Keto Diet Book for Beginners

A guide to understanding the science behind the Ketogenic Diet with proven tips for long-term success and rapid weight loss

Plus a 14-day Meal Plan to Get You Started

Angel Lawal

ISBN: 9798846545939

Contents

Introduction: What is Ketogenic Dieting?

Taking control of your journey towards healthy living can be challenging, but the key to success is implementing effective solutions that are compatible with your lifestyle.

Considering today's flurry of news around diets and health fads, it can be difficult to choose a new and sustainable meal plan for your life. Fortunately, on the ketogenic diet also known as keto, this can be achieved without committing to a lifetime of extreme routines and tasteless meals. In fact, you can meet your health goals by making a few adjustments to what you eat and how you eat. Welcome to the world of keto; a high fat, low carbohydrate diet that retrains the body to burn fat for energy in a process described as ketosis.

Historically, the diet was used to treat patients with poorly-controlled epilepsy, but as new research has emerged, greater health benefits have been discovered. Today, the keto diet is praised for its ability to achieve enhanced weight loss and for its capability to prevent and manage a wide range of health conditions such as heart disease, diabetes, alzheimer's and more.

This book will serve as an introduction for beginners into the keto diet. It contains useful tips and detailed explanations of the latest research into the diet and a 14-day meal plan to get you started. At times you may experience temporary side effects while adjusting to this diet, so to help you along the way, this book will detail what to expect and discuss exactly how you can limit and manage them. It will also provide you with tools to figure out which keto method is best for your lifestyle, so you can easily settle into your new routine. However, this diet is not suitable for everyone, so please speak to your doctor if you are pregnant, breastfeeding, have any medical conditions, a history of eating disorders or have had your gallbladder removed before starting this diet.

The Different Ketogenic Diets

As its popularity has grown, so also has the number of variations on the ketogenic diet. They all follow the same principles, but each variation has its own daily macronutrients ratios and or eating styles. You only need to follow the ratios outlined and fill it with suitable foods you like. Before anything else, remember to work out the total calories you need in a day. This number is different for everyone and will be defined by your gender, activity level and weight goals. The results you get from this diet won't happen overnight; therefore, how well you integrate and maintain these guidelines into your daily life will determine the success achieved. With this in mind, carefully assess each of the keto variations and the changes they require before implementing it into your lifestyle. To avoid choosing a difficult diet that quickly becomes unsustainable, this chapter will show you how to select the keto variation best for you, so you can hit the ground running.

Strict Keto

This version of ketogenic dieting refers to the original and most extreme style of keto. It reduces your overall calories and heavily restricts carbohydrates. It can have accelerated weight loss effects if it is practised carefully alongside an active lifestyle. It is also known as the therapeutic keto diet and was developed to treat seizures in children with epilepsy. Due to the intense nature of its restrictions and its exceedingly low protein intake, this diet is only recommended for those seeking an alternative treatment to seizure medication after speaking with a doctor.

If you are new to ketosis, you should follow a less restrictive plan that makes the adjustment to keto more tolerable. Despite having some popularity within the keto community, it should only be followed temporarily and for short periods at a time. The strict keto diet limits your number of carbohydrates to about 15 to 30 grams a day. For example, a large potato has 20 grams, and a single banana contains 27 grams of carbohydrates. This would mean avoiding bread, pasta and anything high in sugar to maintain your state of ketosis. The macronutrient guideline for the strict keto diet splits your calorie intake into a ratio of 90% fat, 6% protein and only 4% carbohydrates. With most of your diet consisting of fat and low protein levels, the high potential for side effects should be noted.

The bottom line for this version of the diet is that it's an extreme way to achieve the benefits of keto and should be practised with caution. Avoid it if you are not seeking an alternative to anticonvulsant medication. If this diet still appeals to your goals, consider trying it in intermittent phases. This will ensure that you aid your body in its journey towards ketosis while avoiding any risks of nutrient deficiency. If you follow this version, you should also do this alongside the supervision of a doctor or specialist.

Standard Keto

This is an adjusted version of the strict diet that still provides the benefits of ketosis. While it can still be a difficult transition, this version of the diet has been modified to be more accessible for keto newcomers and easier to maintain in the long run. With this version, you can eat slightly more carbohydrates, between 20 to 50 grams a day. This equates to over half a kilogram of keto-friendly vegetables like peppers and tomatoes, but only half of one hamburger bun. Such comparisons are important, as carbohydrates are nearly everywhere but not in the same quantities—this will be explained as we go along. The standard keto diet's macronutrient ratio requires that your daily intake be around 75% fat, 20% protein and 5% carbohydrates. With more protein and a substantial reduction in dietary fat, this style offers a more balanced approach than the strict keto diet.

The standard keto diet can still be a tough transition to make at first, but it promises a balanced routine that helps you reposition your total calorie intake. It maintains the core benefits of ketosis and results in fewer cravings and hunger pangs than the strict keto diet.

Cyclical Keto

This version involves following the standard keto diet for five days, with two days off to significantly increase your carbohydrate intake. These days off are also known as refeeding days and will bring you out of ketosis. This will allow your body to refill its glucose reserves so you can also reap the benefits of having carbohydrates in your diet.

For 5 days, it is recommended that you split your daily calories to 5% of carbohydrates, 75% fats and 20% protein. During the latter 2 days, you need to increase your carbohydrate intake to 50%, leaving protein and fats to each account for 25% of your daily calorie allowance.

The increased carbohydrate flexibility makes this version of the keto diet more sustainable in the long term and ultimately more appealing to the mass market; however, the quality of your carbohydrates should be considered. White bread should be avoided and replaced with foods with good-quality carbohydrates that are also high in vitamins, minerals and fibre, such as sweet potatoes, butternut squash, brown rice, oats, quinoa, beans and lentils.

If you adopt cyclical keto into your lifestyle, consider intermittent fasting and high-intensity workouts as an add-on to aid a quick return to ketosis after your refeeding days.

Targeted Keto

If you are an endurance athlete, the targeted approach to keto may help you achieve better results and improve your overall performance. Recent studies have pointed to a potential increase in endurance and physical capacity when athletes follow this version of the keto diet for about 28 days, and sometimes for as few as 10 days.

To follow this version, you should already be acquainted with ketogenic dieting and have practised it for some time, the recommendation being at least a month. It maintains the standard keto ratio but allows an additional 20 to 30 grams of carbohydrates to be consumed 30 to 45 minutes before or after exercising. This ensures the extra carbohydrates consumed are burned off as energy during your workout to prevent your body leaving ketosis. Essentially this approach works as a pre-workout carbohydrate load that targets periods of intense physical activity.

Following this approach can lead to accelerated weight loss, which can be beneficial for some athletes but not everyone. If you are an experienced athlete who has attempted keto before and wants to see better results, the targeted keto approach could be for you. However, if you follow a low-intensity exercise regime or go to the gym casually, then you should try the standard or cyclical keto version instead.

High-Protein Keto

Whilst the strict version of keto heavily limits your protein intake, increasing your dietary protein won't stop you from achieving a state of ketosis. This high-protein diet is usually aimed at individuals who partake in high levels of exercise and seek to increase their muscle mass. It is also recommended for anyone seeking to prevent muscle breakdown or those with signs of protein deficiency. It follows an adjusted macronutrient ratio which prioritises more protein than any other version of the keto diet. In this version, protein should make up approximately 30% of your total calorie intake, with 65% fat and 5% carbohydrates.

The importance of this high-protein approach is that ketosis can still be achieved despite lower levels of fat consumption. Therefore, all the usual benefits of the keto diet will apply while you build and retain muscle mass. As with all other keto versions, your protein intake must come from varied sources such as beef, fish, lamb, nuts and seeds. Finally, remember to adjust the total number of calories you consume to your weight goals and body requirements.

Lazy Keto

If you are already daunted by calculating your required macronutrient ratios, lazy keto cuts through these complications. In this variation, you only need to track your carbohydrates and stick to eating 50 grams or less per day. This completely removes the need to track your daily calories, protein or fat intake.

Although this form will not be as effective as the carefully planned versions, if you keep your carbohydrate intake low enough, the effects of ketosis may still be noticeable.

While this variation is not as restrictive as the standard forms of keto, you should know the health benefits experienced may not be as expansive or prominent as with the other versions of the diet.

Mediterranean Keto

Many dietitians and doctors praise the benefits of the Mediterranean diet, which focuses on eating heart-healthy foods. In this keto version, you follow the standard keto diet using foods with high nutrient densities from the Mediterranean cuisine. Think of seafood, nuts wholegrains and unsaturated fats, such as avocados and olive oil. The Mediterranean keto diet offers many of the same benefits as the regular Mediterranean diet but with extra benefits that only keto provides. Unlike the standard Mediterranean diet, achieving ketosis is your goal. With this in mind, stick to eating around 50 grams of carbohydrates a day and avoid Mediterranean foods such as bread and starch-heavy tubers such as potatoes and beetroot.

The good thing about this variation of the keto diet is that it may be one of the most heart-healthy approaches to practice keto, as it strictly prescribes followers eat healthy Mediterranean fats.

Keto 2.0

After reading about these keto versions, the restrictive nature of the keto diet might still seem daunting, especially the shift to such low amounts of carbohydrates. Incorporating further variations might be the thing that helps you stick to it. While the high dietary fat might not appeal to everyone, keto 2.0 is gaining some traction. Essentially, it rebalances your macronutrient guidelines to make it more appealing to wider audiences. This keto version encourages you to include whole grains, leaner cuts of meat and legumes into your usual keto diet. It also allows you to add fruits and vegetables higher in carbohydrates, normally avoided in other keto forms. The total fat percentage is decreased from around 70% to 50% of your daily calorie intake, raising your protein up to 30%, and controversially bringing your carbohydrates up to 20% instead of the standard 5%.

Keto 2.0 has been specifically developed to aid your transition into the keto lifestyle, and some experts are also touting it as a maintenance phase for your long-term keto journey.It might sound like an extended version of keto cycling by offering you more carbohydrates daily. The downside is, your body won't stay in ketosis for as long as the other keto forms. This will impact your total weight loss, but the results should still be clear as you carefully select the most nutritious foods to eat. The only caveat with keto 2.0 is that it is very new, and no significant body of research supports it. By looking at its components, however, it is easy to see that keto 2.0 can ease you into one of the more restrictive forms of keto, or even be used as a break if the cravings become too great and you feel tempted to quit.

To summarise, keto 2.0 is closer to a low-carbohydrate diet than to an authentic version of keto. If you struggle to make the changes necessary to enter ketosis, this bridge version can help your body and mind ease into a long-term keto commitment. While it is true that your body is either in ketosis or not, the real trick is in training your body to adjust to the changes so that you can manage your new diet regularly. By transitioning with keto 2.0, you will see an increased chance of sustaining a more restrictive version of keto once your body is ready. It will also result in a significantly lower frequency of cravings and hunger pangs than if you dove straight into the standard keto diet.

Which Keto is Right for you?

Knowing which keto diets right for you will depend on your goals and current lifestyle. Before trying one of the diets, identify the total number of calories you need to achieve your weight or fitness goals and then assess which of the keto versions best match your lifestyle. If you engage in cardiovascular and strength training, you must get lots of heart-healthy protein and eat bigger meal sizes, so the high protein or targeted keto approach may suit you best. All variations on keto can achieve weight loss and increased health benefits, but only if you listen to your body and give it what it needs.

If you feel like combining different elements of each diet, go ahead. By doing so, you can find the perfect rhythm and routine for your keto lifestyle. Accomplishing this will mean that instead of becoming a fad diet only maintained for a few weeks, you can steadily develop and integrate new habits to sustain a long-term health commitment. The only strict guideline for the keto approach is limiting your carbohydrate intake to achieve the coveted ketogenic state; the rest is up to you. But try not to make too many changes as this could slow or possibly stop your progression into ketosis and reduce your chances of gaining the full health benefits of the diet. The next chapter is dedicated to demystifying keto tales and showing you how ketosis can benefit your lifestyle.

Chapter 1
Dispelling Keto Myths

You now have a comprehensive understanding of the different ketogenic diets and how they can help you on your journey to health. You might even have an idea about how you can effectively integrate them into your daily life. Don't worry if this isn't the case. As we debunk some of the more common myths, you will see that keto is easily within your grasp and that these negative presumptions largely stem from the extreme nature of the original and strictest keto diet. Its restrictive nature and low number of calories shocked the public when it was first introduced, and like other modern revisions on dieting, misinformation and rumours have spread ever since. This chapter looks at some of the most enduring keto myths and gives you well-researched answers to understand the truth behind them.

Myth #1: Keto is impossible to maintain

The majority of keto naysayers are quick to mention that it is impossible to stick with it for long periods. Most people will complain about the side effects associated with the diet. Generally, these side effects are temporary and can be managed in several ways, which will be detailed later in this book. You also need to remember that every journey is different, as are attitudes towards keto. Like any serious adjustment to your lifestyle, keto is a long-term commitment. Making these changes can be difficult if you do not anticipate the effort required to follow it through. Mental preparation is as necessary as meal preparation. Making sustainable changes is the most crucial aspect to remember when switching over to the ketogenic lifestyle. These sustainable changes can be anything that helps you stick with your keto commitment. This starts by selecting the keto diet that matches your lifestyle and goals. Remember, each keto version has an acceptable amount of flexibility as long as you limit your carbohydrate intake. This flexibility can involve trying out keto cycling or the lazy version first or even incorporating elements of both into your lifestyle. It would also be wise to steadily transition into your chosen keto diet by starting with a low-carbohydrate diet first, like keto 2.0. This may significantly increase your chances of adjusting to these changes instead of becoming overwhelmed.

In theory, sticking to meal plans and macronutrient guidelines sounds easy, but when you factor in the unpredictability of life, routines can be affected, and you might dip out of ketosis unwillingly.

To avoid this and sustain your ketogenic state long term, you should try to anticipate as many challenges as possible and plan accordingly. Once you have found an adaptable keto routine, this won't be a problem. Whipping out keto-friendly snacks on the go or looking at the restaurant menu for low-carbohydrate meals prior to you going can be the difference between a short- and long-term commitment to ketogenic dieting. You can also minimise the stress of remaining adherent by approaching meal service providers that either deliver the ingredients you need to cook at home or have them prepare the completed meal for you.

Myth #2: No carbohydrates

The "low-carbohydrate, high-fat" slogan that follows the keto diet seems to instil the idea that to achieve ketosis one must avoid carbohydrates altogether. The supposed aim of many weight-loss diets suggests that cutting out carbohydrates entirely will accelerate your weight loss. This is only true in a limited sense. While excessive carbohydrates will result in weight gain, your body needs some carbohydrates to function correctly. If you removed all carbohydrates, you would also have to give up a host of healthy vegetables and forgo herbs, spices, and most oils, restricting yourself to a diet that consists only of animal protein and fat. This is not only unappealing but also potentially harmful to your health. Drastically removing carbohydrates from your diet can impair your immune system's ability to function correctly and take away vital amounts of glucose from the brain, leaving you irritable and tired. You should ensure you eat around 50 grams of carbohydrates a day.

Carbohydrates are found in a wide array of foods, and within those foods, the amount and types of carbohydrates aren't equal. It is important to find nutrient-dense sources of carbohydrates that will fill your plate and stomach without surging your sugar levels. With this in mind, you need to look out for three types of carbohydrates, but only one is important for the keto diet. These are carbohydrates high in fibre, such as avocados, almonds, unsweetened coconut, pistachios, wholegrain pasta. The other carbohydrates are starches, such as white bread, rice, cereals and sugars, which include canned fruit and processed cereals. Both are associated with elevating blood sugar levels and weight gain. Unfortunately for any readers with a sweet tooth, sugary treats and drinks will have to be removed or at the very least, limited within your diet.

Myth #3: Any source of fat is good

Besides the massive reduction in carbohydrates, the other main change in ketogenic dieting is to include high amounts of fatty foods in your diet. Such an increase might spark concern when considering issues such as cholesterol levels and heart disease. However, there are three different types of fat and they are not all equal. Trans fats and saturated fats are known to be harmful to your health; limiting them should be a priority on keto. Trans fats are mostly found in foods cooked in hydrogenated oils, such as deep-fried foods, which raise your low-density lipoprotein (LDL) cholesterol. That's the bad cholesterol known for clogging arteries.

Saturated fats also raise LDL cholesterol, but not to the same level as trans fats. These fats can be found in many of our staple foods, including cheeses and other dairy products, some meats such as bacon and beef, and grain-based baked goods such as biscuits. By avoiding trans fats and limiting saturated fats, you can maintain low amounts of LDL cholesterol and reduce the risk of heart disease. On keto, healthy fats such as mono- and polyunsaturated fats should make up most of your fat consumption. Monounsaturated fats include olive oil, avocados, nuts and seeds, polyunsaturated fats include fish, walnuts and flaxseeds, sunflower and soybean oils. Along with avoiding processed foods and starch-heavy carbohydrates, these good types of unsaturated fats have been shown to lower blood pressure, improve your blood cholesterol levels and reduce your risk of cardiovascular problems. Foods rich in omega-3 fatty acids, such as fish, have been shown to increase mental clarity and greatly aid the body in functioning normally.

Practicing the keto diet requires a new source of energy after you ditch the carbohydrates. While focusing on fat seems to disagree with everything you thought you knew about dieting, your body depends on healthy fats, especially the ones that keep your heart strong and don't clog your arteries. By providing these new, healthy sources of energy, your body can enter ketosis without compromising other areas of your health.

Myth #4: Keto is only for people with chronic illnesses

Despite initially being developed to alleviate the symptoms of epilepsy, keto can be practised by anyone seeking a better quality of life. Its varied benefits mean that for those looking to lose weight, a carefully practised keto diet can help you achieve your results without significantly compromising on the taste of your meals. In addition, this high-fat, low-carbohydrate approach has been linked to preventing common diseases like heart disease and Alzheimer's disease and some forms of cancer. Due to these metabolic mechanisms, some individuals should avoid attempting keto as it may negatively affect some underlying medical conditions. With those with type 1 and type 2 diabetes, specific versions of the keto and low-carbohydrate diets are prescribed. In these instances, careful medical supervision is required. Later, we'll discuss all the potential benefits of keto in preventing disease onset.

Myth #5: Keto is bad for you

A typical headline for keto diets is that they are bad for your health. This is only true if you decide to stick to unhealthy fat sources and forget that there are more protein sources than red meat. Sticking to varied macronutrient sources will help you maintain a healthy balance. Without proper planning, simply limiting carbohydrates will not do the trick as your body needs fresh foods packed full of vitamins and minerals. Unlike a general diet that relies on bread and starch, your body will thank you for filling it with fresh alternatives, such as cauliflower, mushrooms and courgettes. For example, spiralized courgette makes an excellent pasta replacement that consists of fibre, minerals and protein.

When you plan your keto carefully and eat healthy ingredients in line with your body's requirements, you can limit issues with your diet while gaining many of keto's great benefits.

Myth #6: You cannot build muscle on keto

With the restriction of carbohydrates and proteins, there is an assumption you cannot build muscle on a ketogenic diet, but this isn't the case.

Studies have shown that a ketogenic diet can provide strength and performance benefits that can help you build muscle. But to reach this goal, the amount of protein and daily calories you consume must be appropriately calculated.

As a rough guideline, it's estimated that you increase your daily calorie allowance by approximately 10 to 15% to build muscle. For example, the average adult woman requires around 2,000 calories per day, so to build muscle, this would need to be increased by 15%, giving a new total daily calorie allowance of 2,300.

The one essential macronutrient needed to build muscle is protein. However, there are concerns that when the body consumes too much protein, it could create more sugar during digestion, pushing the body out of ketosis. Fortunately, there is a high-protein keto method that works and describes exactly how ketosis can still be maintained even while protein intake is increased. In this method, protein should only account for up to 30% of your total daily calorie consumption, while fat and carbohydrates make up 65% and 5%, respectively.

With this in mind, calculate and monitor your protein and carbohydrate intake to ensure you maintain ketosis whilst building muscle. Your body will rely mostly on fat for fuel, so make sure you also consume enough fats. To make these assessments and calculations easier, I have outlined a formula below:

- First, find out what your daily calorie allowance is for muscle gain.
- Then, multiply this number by 0.3. This will give you your daily protein allowance in calories.
- Similarly, multiply this new total daily calorie allowance by 0.05 to give you the total number of carbohydrates you can consume a day.
- Finally, calculate the amount of fats required by multiplying your total daily calorie allowance by 0.65.
- If you wish to convert your protein and carbohydrate values from calories into grams divide by 4. Likewise, to convert your fat values from calories to grams, divide by 9. This is because approximately 9 calories are present in every 1 gram of fat and 4 calories in every gram of protein and carbohydrates.

To make this even clearer, let's take an example of a female who requires 2,300 calories for muscle gain:

- To calculate her protein intake, multiply 2,300 by 0.3, and you will get a total of 690 calories, equivalent to 30% of her calorie intake. To convert this into grams, divide 690 by 4, to get a sum of 173 grams. This means that 690 calories or 173 grams of protein need to be consumed daily.
- Similarly, 5% of her calorie intake should be carbohydrates. Therefore, multiply 2,300 by 0.05 and this will give 115 calories. To convert this into grams, divide 115 by 4 to give you 29 grams of carbohydrates.

- Finally, fat should account for 65% of her daily calorie consumption, so multiply 2,300 by 0.65, which will give a total of 1,495 calories. Should you wish to convert this into grams, divide 1,495 by 9, and you will get a total of 166 grams of fat.

Therefore, for this individual to build muscle and remain in ketosis, they would need to eat approximately 690 calories of protein, 115 calories of carbohydrates and 1,495 calories of fat in a day. In most cases, the tendency is for people to align with the standard keto diet macronutrient values, but you're likely to find the high-protein keto guidelines provide much better results for muscle gain than the standard keto diet.

Aside from the nutritional aspect, these factors should also be considered:

1. Resistance training must be done at least twice a week to build muscle.
2. Training should involve lifting weights, squats, bench presses, pull-ups, push-ups and strength-based exercises.
3. If you are new to any form of training, it is best to hire a personal trainer to help you effectively reach your goals and reduce your risk of injury.

Chapter 2
A Closer Look at Ketosis

We have touched on some of the metabolic mechanisms of the keto diet, but this chapter goes one step further to ensure you are well informed on the effects ketosis has on the body.

An average person's diet consists largely of carbohydrates. These are found in bread, potatoes, starchy pasta and pastries, not to mention foods and drinks high in sugar. When these foods are broken down, they are converted to glucose and used as an energy source for the body. However, if too many carbohydrates are consumed, the excess glucose produced is stored as glycogen and eventually fats, leading to long-term weight gain. Another downside of eating large amounts of carbohydrate-rich foods is the sugar crash and fatigue you experience after a glucose surge in your bloodstream. Switching to a ketogenic diet and avoiding such refined sugars can help anyone improve their daily energy levels.

As your body loses its dependence on carbohydrates and glucose, it undergoes a new metabolic process known as ketosis to obtain energy. In this process, fats from your diet are broken down to ketones and are used as an energy source to fuel the body.

Remember, this can be a drastic change for your body, and adjusting your carbohydrate intake should be done gradually and carefully. How quickly you achieve the state of ketosis varies from person to person, depending on factors such as previous diet, body weight and level of activity. There are many ways to detect if you have entered ketosis, the most accurate being a ketone urine strip or blood test; other indicators will be highlighted as you read further along this chapter, so simply note how your body feels and compare it against the signs outlined.

The Health Benefits of Ketosis

The keto diet has many health benefits, but one of the most important findings from medical studies is that the source of your daily foods is what matters most. When you select foods like whole grains, plant-derived protein, and heart-healthy fats, your morbidity risk reduces significantly. This chapter will outline these benefits and give possible mechanisms behind them.

Epilepsy

Since the 1920s, the ketogenic diet has been used to reduce seizures in children with poorly-controlled epilepsy—a chronic condition characterised by regular seizures. These seizures result from abnormal electrical discharges firing within the brain. In a clinical study, it was discovered that 25% of epileptic children on the keto diet had fewer seizures, with up to 20% seeing more than a 90% reduction in their seizures. Although the mechanism behind this is still not understood by scientists, what is clear is the unique combination of this high-fat and low-carbohydrate diet alters electrical signalling within the brain thereby reducing its potential to initiate seizures.

Diabetes

The ketogenic diet has also been found to significantly benefit patients with prediabetes and type 2 diabetes. These benefits have included improved management of their blood sugar levels and in some patients a reduction in the use of their medication. Research has shown possible mechanisms behind this phenomenon could be due to the diet's ability to burn excess fat, which has significant links to increasing the body's sensitivity to insulin, a function impaired in this condition. In addition, the reduction of ingested carbohydrates means less glucose is being produced during digestion, resulting in fewer fluctuations in blood sugar levels and better long-term management.

Weight Loss

There are two mechanisms that keto employs to promote weight loss. The first is to boost metabolism and the second is to reduce appetite. The first mechanism occurs during ketosis when fat stores are depleted to produce energy. This depletion causes less fat to be stored in the body and results in an overall reduction in body weight.

The second mechanism comes into play through the system that regulates our appetite. Typically, when calories are lowered during a weight-loss program, hunger hormones are released, which trigger an increase in food intake.

However, on keto, the elevated fat levels cause you to feel fuller for longer, resulting in a reduced appetite. This feeling may also be due to the ketones released, as they play a role in stabilising your blood sugar levels and inhibiting the hunger hormones release.

As a result, rapid weight loss is a classic sign your body is in ketosis.

Improved Heart Health

Low-density lipoprotein (LDL) threatens your cardiovascular system. In high levels, LDL causes blockages in the arteries, cutting off vital blood supply to the heart, while high-density lipoprotein (HDL) does the opposite and prevents blockages.

The healthy fats you consume on a ketogenic diet improve your health by reducing bad cholesterol and increasing good cholesterol within the body. This was proved within a 2017 study on the keto diet, which demonstrated significant reductions in LDL with notable increases in HDL levels among people on the diet. Interestingly, another study involving a group of men showed that 22 out of 26 biomarkers for cardiovascular disease decreased within 6 weeks of starting the diet. This is important as this reduction in your LDL cholesterol and cardiovascular disease biomarkers leads to a lower risk of heart disease and stroke, both of which are common causes of premature death and disability in the UK. This suggests that following the keto diet with the right food choices could improve your heart health in the short term and prevent health complications in the long run.

Protection of Brain Function

While the brain prefers to use glucose as its primary energy source, it can also use ketones to function. With ketones becoming the predominant energy source, studies suggest it can boost the brain's energy levels by up to 75%. This leaves the small carbohydrates allowed in the diet to sustain the parts of the brain that require only glucose to function.

In neurological disorders, such as Alzheimer's and Parkinson's disease, the keto diet is also beneficial. Although it is unclear how ketones protect the brain, health experts suggest ketones' antioxidant, and anti-inflammatory effects together with its ability to provide extra energy to brain cells may be possible pathways. In these three ways, it appears that a ketogenic diet can help prevent diseases that attack the tissue in the brain. Additionally, this diet has been shown to decrease the risk of nerve cell damage in the brain by preventing the overstimulation of a dominant neurotransmitter known as glutamate.

Reduction of Chronic Fatigue Syndrome

The mitochondria serve as the energy production site, or powerhouse, of your cells so your body can function. A chemical is released called adenosine triphosphate (ATP) and the higher the levels of ATP, the higher your energy levels will be. Conversely, when ATP levels are low, this can result in chronic fatigue syndrome, a long-term condition characterised by extreme tiredness. ATP is manufactured when the mitochondria combine glucose from food with oxygen from the air we breathe.

When you are in ketosis, glucose is not readily available, so your body breaks ketones down to form the energy source, ATP. During this process, more ATP molecules are generated than with a glucose output. This increase in ATP means you can experience a marked increase in energy levels and a subsequent decrease of the symptoms displayed in chronic fatigue syndrome. Therefore, an increase in energy is another great sign that your body has entered ketosis.

Increased Antioxidants

On the keto diet, there is an increased level of antioxidants produced. These antioxidants help to decrease cell damage by maintaining the levels of free radicals within the body.

When the levels of free radicals become higher than that of antioxidants a state of oxidative stress is reached. This state can have detrimental effects on your DNA and can result in cell death that leads to illnesses such as heart disease, cancer and diabetes.

As the body is constantly forming free radicals, it is critical a supply of antioxidants is produced to counteract its effect. Fortunately, ketosis triggers an increase in the antioxidant glutathione, which keeps free radicals balanced & protects our cells against damage.

You can also incorporate more antioxidants into your body through the types of foods you eat on the ketogenic diet.

One rich source of antioxidants is turmeric, which also acts as an anti-inflammatory agent, lowering inflammation and its related pain. Fruits and vegetables containing high levels of vitamin A, C and E also have highly effective antioxidants. Other food sources rich in antioxidants include

- vitamin supplements
- lean red meat
- fish
- green tea
- pecans
- berries
- artichokes
- kale
- red cabbage
- spinach
- dark chocolate

Therefore, by going on the keto diet and incorporating antioxidant-rich vegetables and food sources in your meal plans, you can increase your levels of antioxidants and naturally protect your body from many illnesses.

Chapter 3
Keto Drawbacks and How to Avoid Them

The journey to ketosis can be a dramatic change for your body, especially when you suddenly restrict certain foods in ways that your body isn't used to. As your body changes the way it obtains energy, don't be surprised if you experience side effects along the way.

Hunger Pangs and Cravings

An adjustment to the keto diet could result in a dramatic increase in appetite known as hunger pangs or cravings. This typically occurs at the beginning of the diet when the body has no glucose stores left and isn't effectively burning fats for energy. As a result, hunger signals are sent to the brain to replenish these glucose stores.

However, hunger pangs are short-term and to limit their effects, the key is to ensure you reach and maintain a state of ketosis. This can be achieved by eating the recommended macronutrient ratios for your chosen keto diet, incorporating intermittent fasting and exercising regularly.

Once your body is using ketones as its main energy source, hunger pangs should subside. This should typically only take a week or two, but if you are struggling with it, try a slow adjustment into the keto diet, with a low-carb diet like keto 2.0. If your hunger pangs continue after two weeks, seek the professional advice of your GP or a licensed nutritionist.

Keto Flu and Keto Breath

Keto flu

Some people who go on the keto diet experience keto flu. These symptoms usually take place about a week after starting the diet, but will typically resolve once the body adjusts to using ketones as its main energy source.

Symptoms

Some symptoms that can be experienced are a headache, foggy brain, fatigue, irritability, nausea, sleeping difficulties and constipation. If these symptoms persist for more than a few days, or they have an adverse effect on your daily life, you should take a break from the diet and speak to your doctor before continuing with it.

Causes

No one knows for sure why the body reacts in this way, but a possible reason could be due to the detoxification process in your body. Alternatively, it could be a reaction to the changes in your gut microbiomes or a form of withdrawal from carbohydrates.

Treatment

The recommended treatment for the keto flu is to drink plenty of water, eat more often during the day and try to increase your intake of colourful vegetables as they are filled with nutrients. Finally, ease slowly into the keto diet to give your body a chance to adjust.

Keto Breath

Keto breath is different to halitosis, also known as bad breath, and is often described as a metallic taste with a scent similar to acetone. Though it can be embarrassing, it is only temporary.

Fatty acids are converted to the ketones hydroxybutyrate, acetoacetate and acetone during ketosis. Acetone is the same ingredient used in nail polish remover. These ketones are removed from the body in the air you exhale and through urination.

Consequently, a classic indication that you've reached ketosis is when your breath smells like nail polish remover or in some cases, fruity.

Treatment

There are a few ways to minimise or eliminate keto breath:

1. Drink more water, as ketones can be flushed out of your system through urination.
2. Eat less protein—when excess protein is broken down, ammonia is produced, which also has a strong odour.
3. Display good oral hygiene—even brushing and flossing your teeth twice a day may not eliminate the keto breath, but it will help to lessen the smell.
4. Mask the odour—you could use sugar-free mints or chewing gum. Be aware that these contain small amounts of carbohydrates which could affect your ketosis state.
5. Be patient—keto breath is temporary and will typically subside as your body adjusts to a lower carbohydrate intake which may take a couple of weeks.

Whilst the likes of keto flu and keto breath aren't appealing, you may notice these side effects are nowhere near as dramatic or severe as they sound. You might come to see them as slight disadvantages compared to your newfound weight loss and high levels of energy.

Weight Cycling or Yo-yoing

Arguably, the one aspect of keto dieting to be aware of is the possibility of weight cycling. This refers to the phenomenon where you suddenly regain the weight you have lost, and it can happen when you lose a lot of fluid weight in the first few days of your diet. It can be quickly regained if you overindulge or decide to spend prolonged periods off your keto diet. You might feel your old cravings come back and can easily revert to processed and carbohydrate-rich foods. These changes may be dangerous for your health as the constant cycling in weight puts stress on your heart and the rest of your cardiovascular system. That is why keto is an entire lifestyle commitment and will require patience to see the best results.

The best way to avoid weight cycling is to opt for a version of the keto diet that suits you to avoid overindulging or relapsing. It will also help if you can slowly incorporate your chosen keto methods into your lifestyle.

Digestive Challenges

When starting the ketogenic journey, a significant change in your diet can lead to common digestive issues like diarrhoea or constipation. As soon as your body has adjusted to your new diet, these symptoms should pass; however, there are a few things you can do to help minimise or overcome these effects. Firstly, keep a note of the foods that have had the most pronounced effects on your digestion. Secondly, increase your intake of low-carbohydrate vegetables high in fibre. Great examples of this include broccoli, red bell peppers, asparagus and mushrooms. Lastly, ensure that you diversify the foods you eat; this will not only decrease the risk of digestive issues but also reduce nutrient deficiencies on the diet.

Ketoacidosis

Ketoacidosis is when the body produces high levels of ketone acids when burning fats. This can result in your blood becoming too acidic and can lead to liver, kidney and brain damage. Those with diabetes are more prone to this, so it is vital to embark on the keto diet after consultations with your doctor if you have this condition.

To prevent ketoacidosis, monitor your blood ketone levels and do not exceed the recommended macronutrient ratios. During nutritional ketosis, it is normal for non-diabetics to have blood ketone levels of 0.5 to 3.0 mmol/L, so make sure that you remain within this range. Also ensure that you watch out for the classic symptoms of ketoacidosis; these include excessive thirst, confusion, frequent urination as well as nausea and vomiting.

If ketoacidosis is not treated, it can be very detrimental to your health, so ensure you check your blood ketone levels regularly, especially if you have diabetes.

Chapter 4
Tips and Tricks for a Successful Keto

Achieving a state of ketosis can be a rewarding experience with various health and lifestyle benefits, but adapting to a keto routine will take time and effort. Remember to carefully plan your transition and adjust your carbohydrate intake gradually as you progress. Firstly, consider your current mindset and eating habits. Think about how you can overcome them? How can you effectively make this switch and commit to it? Fortunately for you, this chapter will provide you with the best tips and tricks that you'll need to turn keto into a lifestyle.

Keto-Friendly and Keto-Avoidant

To start you off, a comprehensive list of the best and worst ingredients for your keto diet has been outlined to help you stick to a ketogenic diet and find delicious foods for an everyday approach. These suggestions will help you fill in any gaps in your meal plan as well as give you interesting ideas on how to snack in a keto-friendly manner.

Protein

The most common sources of protein are meat, poultry and fish. They contain little to no carbohydrates with a good supply of fat, depending on the meat.

Fish such as salmon, sardines, mackerel and other fatty fish are rich in omega-3, linked to improved cognitive health. Salmon also contains high amounts of vitamin B, potassium and selenium. To gain the best benefits, it is recommended that you have fish or shellfish at least twice a week. Ideal meats that can be consumed on the keto diet are steak, ham, sausage and turkey.

Eggs are a versatile and healthy source of protein. One large egg contains approximately 1 gram of carbohydrates and 6 grams of protein. Although egg yolks are high in cholesterol, research shows they don't raise your blood cholesterol as foods high in trans and saturated fats do. But if you're still worried about cholesterol, you can cook with egg whites instead.

A vegan or vegetarian protein variant can be avocados, nuts and seeds. Plain Greek yoghurt, as well as cottage cheese, is also protein-rich. However, they do contain some carbohydrates. A portion of 122 grams of yoghurt contains 4 grams of carbohydrates and 9 grams of protein. The same amount of cottage cheese will contain 5 grams of carbohydrates and 11 grams of protein. You can either have it as a stand-alone snack or mix it with chopped nuts, cinnamon or other spices.

Oils and Fats

The fats encouraged on the keto diet are unsaturated fats. These fat sources have positive effects on your health, including improved blood cholesterol levels and reduced risk of cardiovascular disease.

Unsaturated fats are split into two groups: monounsaturated and polyunsaturated fats. Examples of monounsaturated fats include olive oil, avocados, pumpkins and nuts such as almonds, hazelnuts and pecans. Polyunsaturated fats are found in sunflower, corn, soybean, flaxseed oils, and included in walnuts and fish.

Other foods rich in fat are cream and butter, but moderate consumption of high-fat dairy products is required.

Eating coconut oil is also great whilst on the keto diet as it contains fats called medium-chain triglycerides (MCT). These fats are quickly taken to the liver, readily converted to ketones and used for energy. This is beneficial in helping you to achieve ketosis quickly. However, introduce coconut oil slowly into your diet as it could induce stomach cramps and diarrhoea.

Fruit

Avocados are fruits rich in several minerals and vitamins. Though they have a high carbohydrate level, over 75% of it comprises fibre, so in an avocado containing 9 grams of carbohydrates, 7 grams of this is fibre, leaving 2 grams as net carbohydrates. An avocado a day can have great benefits on your cardiovascular system, and it can lower your levels of LDL cholesterol.

Berries are low in carbohydrates and high in fibre, making them the perfect companion to a ketogenic diet. They're also loaded with antioxidants which reduce inflammation and protect against diseases.

Olives have the same health benefits as the oil and contain anti-inflammatory properties that help prevent cell damage. Olives may vary in carbohydrate content due to their varied size, but their carbohydrate content is generally low as half of it comprises fibre.

Other keto-friendly fruits include watermelons, strawberries, raspberries, blueberries, lemons, tomatoes, peaches and cantaloupes.

Vegetables

It is best to stick to non-starchy vegetables such as asparagus, baby corn, bean sprouts and mushrooms, which are also high in nutrients. They contain fibre needed in a low-carbohydrate diet, and have antioxidants that protect you against cell damage.

Kale, broccoli and cauliflower have been linked to a decrease in cancer and heart disease risk. These vegetables are also suitable substitutes for high-carbohydrate foods. For example, cauliflower can replace rice, mashed potatoes or even pizza bases. Courgettes and squash can also replace spaghetti.

Other vegetables ideal for keto are cabbage, cucumber, aubergines, lettuce, peppers, spinach and red cabbage.

Dairy Products

Cheese is low in carbohydrates but high in saturated fats, so it must be eaten in moderation within the keto diet to avoid increasing your risk of cardiovascular disease. On the plus side, it's a great source of protein and calcium, which is beneficial for building muscle and supporting your bone growth and development.

Cheeses compatible with the ketogenic diet are unprocessed cheeses like blue cheese, cheddar, cottage cheese, feta, goat's cheese, mozzarella and cream cheese.

Nuts and Seeds

Nuts are healthy as they are high in unsaturated fat and low in carbohydrates. Eating nuts can help reduce the risk of heart disease, certain cancers, depression and chronic diseases. Nuts are also rich in fibre, making you feel full and absorb fewer calories. The carbohydrates will vary among the different nuts.

The suggested nuts on the keto diet are almonds, Brazil nuts, cashews, macadamia nuts, pecans, pistachios and walnuts.

Seeds are also a great source of fibre and filled with vital minerals, vitamins and nutrients. They reduce bowel issues and promote heart health. These seeds can be used as part of salads to flavour them or as snacks. They can also be a substitute for bread crumbs when cooking.

Preferred seeds are chia, flax, pumpkin and sesame.

Drinks

Water is the healthiest option for keto-friendly beverages, as it contains no carbohydrates, calories, or additives. There are various flavours available and it is versatile enough to add fruit for extra flavour.

These next set of beverages are also keto-appropriate and contain less than 5 grams of carbohydrates.

Hot drinks:

Several hot drinks are keto-friendly, but you must be aware of what is added to them. Favourable additives include double whipped cream, unsweetened plant-based creams, sweeteners and sugar-free flavouring syrup. Avoid carbohydrate additives such as regular milk, sweetened creamers, sugars and honey.

Black or green tea is a natural option whether you drink it hot or cold. There is usually 1 gram of carbohydrates in a 240-millilitre cup. Black tea is made of aged leaves and has a more robust flavour and darker colour because of its higher caffeine content. Green tea is made from fresh leaves with a more floral flavour, lighter colour and less caffeine.

Coffee is carbohydrate-free, hot or cold. Coffee has a high caffeine content, which boosts your metabolism. It's also a source of chlorogenic acid, an antioxidant that neutralises free radical cells and assists in weight loss.

Cold drinks:

Sparkling water is available in several flavours and is a low-carbohydrate choice. Like water, you can add extra flavour and sweetness to it with limes, while keeping your carbohydrate count low at 1 to 5 grams per serving.

Fruit juice should be avoided as most juices are loaded with sugar. There are exceptions, such as lemon or lime juice, that can be added to water or iced tea. They are low in carbohydrates but hold a lot of flavour. Freshly pressed juices are as susceptible to a high sugar content due to the high level of natural sugars found in fruit.

Vegetable juices are low in carbohydrates and the best vegetables to juice are celery, cucumber, kale or spinach. Store-bought juice might contain added sugar or carbohydrates, and may contain over 10 grams of carbohydrates per serving.

Milk alternatives need to be considered because cow's milk is not recommended for keto as it contains natural sugars. Plant-based milk, including almond milk, coconut milk, macadamia milk and flaxseed milk are great alternatives because of their low carbohydrate content. They are great for drinking, pouring or cooking. It is necessary to be vigilant as some could be sweetened, which is not conducive to the ketogenic diet.

Hard liquors that are naturally carbohydrate-free include vodka, whiskey, rum and tequila. It is often the beverages they are mixed with that make them carbohydrate-heavy as they are often loaded with sugars. It would be best to drink the liquor with zero-sugar mixers like diet coke.

Calculating and Tracking Your Macronutrients

Learning how to track your macronutrients is the number one method to ensure that you achieve ketosis and maintain its benefits. While it may seem daunting to calculate each of your macronutrients and plan your meals, it will become easier with practice. Before you know it, tracking your macros will become second nature, and you can tell what is in the food you eat.

For example, if your target is to consume 2,000 calories per day and you follow a standard keto diet, then your daily calorie consumption should follow the macronutrient ratios of 75% fat, 15 to 20% protein and 5 to 10% carbohydrates. With this in mind, 75% of fat would mean you are to consume roughly 1,500 calories of fat, 495 calories worth of protein and 100 calories of carbohydrates.

As highlighted in previous chapters, carbohydrates and protein yield 4 calories per gram and fat 9 calories per gram. Therefore, to calculate how much 1,500 calories of fat is in grams, divide by 9, which would equal 167 grams of fat. Similarly, to convert 495 calories of protein and 100 calories of carbohydrates into grams, divide both numbers by 4 and you get an answer of 124 grams of protein and 25 grams of carbohydrates.

Once you have worked out approximately how many macronutrients you need a day, you can keep track of it by reading the nutritional labels on your food packaging. Alternatively, you can source this information by downloading digital apps like My Fitness Pal, which have nutritional information for a variety of foods. These aids can also help you to monitor your daily allowance and track your progress against your goals.

Net Carbohydrates Versus Total Carbohydrates

As discussed, your new keto diet will still contain carbohydrates. You should aim to eat healthy sources of carbohydrates with even greater amounts of fibre. In the instance of avocados, they contain 9 grams of total carbohydrate, which consist of starch, fibre and sugars. However, as 7 grams of this comprises fibre, it leaves a net carbohydrate value of 2 grams. Consequently, total carbohydrates are defined as the number of non-fibre and fibre sources of carbohydrates present in a food or meal. But your net carbohydrates only refer to the non-fibre sources, i.e., starch and sugar, as this is the only carbohydrates your body can digest into glucose. With this in mind, it's the value of net carbohydrates you consume a day that needs to be around 50 grams to maintain ketosis. Fortunately, UK nutritional labels display carbohydrates as net carbohydrates and show fibre separately, so it's easy to calculate your macronutrients.

Plan Your Meals Ahead of Time

Taking the time to plan your meals allows you to calculate your carbohydrates, fats and proteins in leisure. This gives you more control over what you eat and allows you to plan the days when you will increase your carbohydrate intake and coordinate it with your training days.

Planning your meals also means you have more time in the week to focus on different forms of training that will allow you to build muscle, lose weight and stay healthy. It allows you to monitor your progress and your emotional and physical well-being. You will also have a clear idea of when to adjust your carbohydrate or protein levels, and if you are still in ketosis.

However, meal prep can be very time-consuming and should be done on a day when your daily commitments are at their lowest. Usually, you can freeze diced or sliced vegetables as well as pre-cut meat and fish into individual portions.

The best way to track if your planning is on par is on a visible platform that is accessible, such as a calendar against the fridge or on the inside of a cupboard door. Meal journals track more than your meals. They give clarity about which foods made you feel good. Try to make your journal fun and exciting as you go, adding notes about interesting new flavours and ideas while trying your new meal plan.

Mind Over Matter

If you can shift your thinking, then changing to a healthier you can be much simpler. Once you have created an image in your head of where you want to be, the next step is manifesting it and keeping yourself motivated. Motivation can be maintained by incorporating regular weigh-in days to check your progress across your journey, taking progress pictures and videos, having positive words of affirmation or booking a holiday in advance to keep you focused on getting in shape. The important thing is finding what that motivation is and maintaining it.

It may also be useful to picture your daily allowance of carbohydrates with all the reliable and healthy sources of food you can replace your sugary and starchy carbohydrates with to make staying in ketosis easier.

Supplementing Your Diet

Similar to vegetarian and vegan diets, when limiting certain sources of protein and other minerals, you must take certain multivitamins and supplements to ensure that your body can function at its best. As a quick guide, certain dietary supplements are great for any diet and person. These include folic acid, omega-3 fatty acids and multivitamins. These general examples contribute to healthy skin and organ tissue, mental focus and better sleep quality. Going to your local retail pharmacy and assessing their individual and general supplements stock will ensure that you are at your healthiest.

In terms of keto-specific supplements, medium-chain triglyceride (MCT) oil can help you produce ketones more quickly and reach your required intake of fatty acids. Largely extracted from coconut oil, MCT oil has become exceedingly popular in health and wellness circles. Studies have shown that part of its effect is to increase the amount of hormones that make you feel full after a meal. This oil is commonly available to purchase at Holland & Barrett.

Cyclical Keto

This process involves following a standard ketogenic diet for five days, followed by a higher-carbohydrate diet for two days; this consistently brings your body in and out of ketosis on a set schedule. The days when you increase your carbohydrate consumption and come out of ketosis will effectively refill your glucose stores. This increases readily-available energy, allowing your muscles and body to work harder during exercise routines and this can be a great add-on to achieving more success with keto.

Who Benefits

If you are an athlete or like to partake in high-intensity workouts, you will find that cyclical keto can benefit you when you need to boost your performance. If the thought of drastically cutting down on your carbohydrates seems daunting or unrealistic to maintain, cyclical keto is helpful because for a set time, you can take in a larger amount of carbohydrates, which could help you stick with the keto diet long-term and fit in better with your social routines.

Who Won't Benefit

If you have previously relapsed with cyclical keto or struggle with self-control when it comes to food, you shouldn't experiment as it may be easy to consume too many calories on refeeding days.

Sometimes, you might be tempted to use carbohydrates with a high sugar content like cake, ice cream and sodas instead of healthy carbohydrates such as beans or lentils. This could counteract the weight-loss benefits of the keto diet, so it's important to have good self-control and indulge in the right carbohydrates such as sweet potatoes, butternut squash, brown rice or oats during these off days.

Intermittent Fasting

Intermittent fasting can accelerate your weight loss on the keto diet and improve your general sense of well-being. It's a period of calorie restriction where you avoid normal food consumption for set periods, including snacking. These restrictions don't include beverages with little to no calories, such as water or black coffee. However, keep an eye on your caffeine intake as fasting with too much coffee can result in jitteriness and anxiety.

In metabolic terms, fasting refers to a state where your body is no longer fed. This means it is not digesting any food and your stomach is empty. Intermittent fasting is deliberate and planned to encourage your body to adapt to a new way of processing food. If you simply skip meals here and there, your body will store fat since it believes food is scarce. So, if you choose to implement fasting into your keto diet, then you must do so with a routine in mind. To be effective, you must maintain a regular fasting routine for at least two weeks to see results.

The great thing about intermittent fasting is it can be adjusted and suited to your daily routine to ensure it doesn't hinder your progress. Once your body has grown accustomed to these fasting periods, it learns to burn fat fast, allowing your body to become extra efficient at utilising its energy potential.

Intermittent fasting might be easier for those who already feel inclined to skip breakfast or lunch during their busy day. Others might find this restriction more challenging, especially since snacking is off the table during a fast. Incorporating and maintaining a routine of intermittent fasting may initially be difficult, but with time and effort, you will see your cravings shrink and your focus sharpen. Below are popular methods of intermittent fasting which can be integrated into your ketogenic diet regime.

The 16/8 Method

This method is the most popular version and is widely discussed and practised by everyone from amateur athletes to health experts. As its name suggests, it breaks your periods of fasting and non-fasting into segments of 16 and 8 hours, respectively.

By fasting for 16 hours a day and only eating during an 8-hour window, you can train your body to cut down on its storage of fat quickly and effectively. If you incorporate the time you spend sleeping into this period, then you can fast without even noticing it. For example, if you eat dinner at 6 p.m. and have a slightly later breakfast at 10 a.m. the next day, you can easily create a 16-hour fast. From 10 am until 6 pm, you can eat and snack on keto-friendly foods all you want, so long as it fits in with your macronutrient guide and your total daily calorie consumption. This shows how easy it can be to incorporate fasting into your routine with no effort. Hunger pangs and urges to snack will steadily diminish as your metabolism adjusts to your fasts, so it's worth implementing this method into your routine before starting the keto diet. These changes to your metabolism can make the transition to keto easier as your body will have already prepared itself for the reduction in calories and restricted mealtimes. You should also consider how you might fit your keto meals into the 8 hours, but this is entirely up to you and will vary depending on your goals.

Only try this method if you feel confident in your ability to forgo food for such long periods. If this extended fasting period proves too difficult, try one of the other methods. They might prove easier for adjusting your total intake.

The 5:2 Method

If weight loss is highest on your list of priorities, then the 5:2 method of fasting can help you reach your goals quickly and effectively. Similar to the 16:8 fasting method, this version splits your week into periods of eating and fasting. By relying on a distinct ratio, it helps you find a routine where your body can adjust to particular periods of reduced calories.

For five days, you need to stick to your regular keto diet, making sure to keep your calories at a level that provides enough nutrients to support your system. You should eat three balanced meals daily and snack on keto-friendly treats in between. For the remaining two days of your week, it's time to limit your calorie intake to about 500 or 600 calories a day, or a suitable low number that fits your macronutrient guideline. This number will vary depending on your gender and fitness goals. Men should stick to no more than 600 calories on these fasting weekends; for women, approximately 500 calories works best.

These two days of heavily reduced calories allow your body to leave the fed state for prolonged periods, making sure that it is able to burn fat fast. On these days, your meals can be divided into two plates of about 250 or 300 calories. Snacking can help sustain you on these fast days but make sure to redistribute your intake accordingly and not add extra calories. This would mean eating smaller meals with slight and careful snacking in between to ensure you don't exceed your calorie allowance.

In place of fasting every day, this method might be easier for some to implement, especially if you are prone to snacking. When incorporating keto into fasting, plan your cheat days before or after your two days of calorie restriction. This can help you weather the hunger pangs while keeping your body in ketosis. If you accidentally cheat on your keto diet, then a period of fasting can help your body reenter ketosis quickly.

Keto and Exercise

At its core, keto helps your body optimize its metabolic processes and combined with regular exercise; its effects are significantly enhanced. This is because being active not only aids a faster progression into ketosis, but it also shares similar health benefits to keto. A prime example of this is weight loss. Keto and exercise can achieve weight loss individually, but when combined, the results are more prominent and quickly achieved. In addition, exercise comes with benefits outside of keto, such as an improved mood and better sleep, which are great bonuses that you can enjoy as part of your new lifestyle.

However, carbohydrates are typically preferred for high-intensity activities like sprinting, boxing and swimming, so following a low-carbohydrate diet might not seem beneficial to some. You can overcome this by increasing your carbohydrate intake before engaging in a high-intensity workout. This can be achieved through either keto cycling or preferably through following the targeted keto diet.

Remember that although exercise increases ketone production and facilitates a quick progression into ketosis, it may take up to 4 weeks for your body to adapt to using it as its primary fuel. Therefore, it is likely that during this time, physical performance may be reduced temporarily.

In the meantime, there are a variety of low-intensity activities that you can incorporate into your routine, such as walking, light jogging and yoga, to keep you going. Be assured that once you've found your rhythm and integrated exercise into your diet, you're on track to living a better-quality life.

Chapter 5
Eating out—Keto-Style

Since so many fast-food outlets and prepackaged foods contain excessive carbohydrates and trans fats, it's easy to imagine why eating out doesn't sound keto-friendly. There are ways around this, and it's not impossible to find exciting new ways to experience your fast-food favourites.

The most important part of learning how to eat out in a smart, keto way is to know your macronutrient consistencies and develop a sixth sense for net carbohydrates when you dine out. Understanding where the carbohydrates come from can ensure that your next coffee or dinner date won't bring you out of ketosis. For example, an average 475-millilitre cappuccino contains a whopping 13 grams of carbohydrates and 130 calories altogether. It does mean that if you have met your total of carbohydrates for the day, opt for a glass of water or black coffee instead. Many restaurants and some fast-food outlets have begun offering healthier alternatives on their menus, but remember that your intake of fast-foods should be kept to a minimum. A diet that consists of mostly fast and processed foods will lead to an increased risk of morbidity and weight gain.

There are absolute rules when dining out. Sugary, carbonated drinks should be avoided and replaced with low-sugar alternatives. This goes for milkshakes and juices too, as their high sugar content is a definite keto sin. It is best to go for water or coffee and tea with no dairy milk or sugar. Besides what you drink, the traditional sides that come with your restaurant meals need to be adjusted. This includes rice and chips, which should be replaced with side salads and roasted vegetables.

Comparing Your Fast Favourites

If you consider some of the most popular takeaways, the number of trans fats and carbohydrates can result in unwelcome weight gain. These highly processed foods are also behind the fatigue and mental fog you may be experiencing.

While it's important to find foods you can indulge in, it's entirely possible to find foods that are delicious and dense in essential nutrients when eating out. Remember that if you cannot find alternatives to your favourites at restaurants, you can always try to make them at home, with fresh, keto-friendly ingredients.

You have the option of *pizza*. Some places offer a keto-friendly version by substituting the flour in their bases for flaxseed, egg, cauliflower or cheese dough. This means that gluten is eliminated, and the carbohydrates in the pizza can be reduced to less than 6 grams. These can be topped with some keto favourites such as mozzarella cheese, bacon, cherry tomatoes, mushrooms, spinach or a tomato sauce. You can also replace the above-mentioned bases with flour made from almonds or coconut.

Fish is always a good choice, especially if it's grilled or steamed. Try to avoid other condiments with it as they have a high sugar and carbohydrate content. Rather, choose mayonnaise, hollandaise sauce or mustard.

Burgers can also be an option as there are places that offer a low-carbohydrate bun version or where this is unavailable, you can ask for the buns to be removed. The filling can be high-protein-based, especially if it has patties, cheese, lettuce, olives and other sauces besides the general condiments.

Grilled or steamed *chicken* needs to be adhered to if you choose that for your meal. Your personal fat requirement will determine which portion of the chicken you will eat. The best option, especially for takeaway, is to have the chicken wrapped in lettuce leaves with a mayonnaise or Hollandaise sauce.

Kebabs are ideal as part of the Mediterranean version of the keto diet. They are usually a good protein-filled option. You need to ensure that their basting sauce is not a generic BBQ sauce, which could contain high carbohydrate and sugar levels.

The spices, legumes and the way the food is prepared make *Indian* cuisine ideal for the ketogenic diet. Using aubergines is widely known, and this vegetable is one with the least carbohydrates—6 grams in a 100-gram serving. Another favourite is paneer, an Indian cheese made from curdled milk and fruit or vegetable acids such as lemon juice. A 100-gram serving of paneer only has less than 4 grams of carbohydrates.

Find or eat *Chinese* dishes steamed or boiled and contain mostly meat, eggs and or non-starchy vegetables. This cuisine often offers a protein-rich selection, as well as steamed or stir-fried vegetables, which can ensure you stay in ketosis without worrying about straying from the diet.

Though it may seem challenging to eat out while on the keto diet, the major task is to know which foods are rich in carbohydrates, and replace them with items that are protein- or fat-rich and choose salads rather than chips. It also means avoiding pairing your meals up with sugar-laden beverages, choosing a flavoured water, or coffee with double cream instead.

Finding alternatives to your favourite takeaways will make your keto journey much easier and more sustainable. However, this will take some research, but doing so could allow you to discover hidden gems in your local area.

Social Strategies While on Keto

At first glance at the keto restrictions, it may feel as though you'll need to turn down invitations to dinner with friends or not attend certain functions if you follow the ketogenic lifestyle- but this isn't the case. You'll still be able to enjoy a social life that includes brunch with the family, a night on the town with friends, or a date with that special someone with the social strategies highlighted in this section. With planning and discipline, you'll see that you don't have to lock yourself in your house.

Happy Hour

Drinks with colleagues are possible when there are several low-carbohydrate options to choose from, including alcoholic beverages. Preferable options are wine and liquor. As a recommendation, a glass or two of dry red wine is suitable and can include Cabernet Sauvignon, Merlot or Pinot Noir. Dry white wine options are Champagne, Chardonnay, Pinot Grigio or Sauvignon Blanc. Liquors like gin, vodka, tequila or whisky can be consumed as these have a carbohydrate content of fewer than 5 grams. Try to avoid mixers like coke, lemonade, tonic water or fruit juices as these often have a high sugar content that could take you out of ketosis. Instead, replace these with sugar-free mixers such as diet coke.

Beer has a high carbohydrate content so it should be avoided. However, there are low-carbohydrate beer versions available that you can request at the bar to avoid stifling your progression to ketosis.

Brunch

Fortunately, many dishes served at brunch are keto-friendly as they contain high amounts of protein. These would include eggs, bacon, sausage, steak, stuffed mushrooms, ham, cheese and smoothies. Be sure to choose water and tea or coffee that is unsweetened as a beverage.

Work Lunches

The best option is to prepare your own lunch for the day, but often having lunch is a means of team building and friendship. You can do several things to prepare for an afternoon with colleagues.

The first is to look at the menu options online beforehand, as this will give you more control over what you can eat. Be aware that when an option says gluten-free, it does not necessarily mean it is keto-friendly. Ask about whether a menu item has sugar or grains.

Base your meals around a protein-filled menu, which could include eggs, steak, cheese or salmon, as these are filled with healthy fats. Dress your salad with olive oil and vinegar. Swap a meal item for a keto alternative. When ordering your entrée, swap your rice for salad or steamed vegetables, or build a meal from the appetisers and sides section of the menu.

Backyard Barbecues

It is hard to resist temptation when attending barbecues, especially when socialising with friends and family. Your options are varied as many foods prepared at a barbecue are protein-based, such as sausage, brisket, smoked chicken and grilled fish. Alternate the regular condiments with keto-friendly sauces like mustard and mayonnaise.

Buffet

A buffet offers various keto-friendly options that can range from a variety of salads, steamed vegetables, grilled seafood and an assortment of meats high in protein. Avoid starchy vegetables, which could consist of potatoes or parsnips. Try to use sauces high in fats and proteins and low in carbohydrates. Alternate salad dressing with lime, lemon juice or olive oil. Select desserts low in carbohydrates, varying from fresh gluten-free tarts, peanut butter pudding or sugar-free chocolate truffles.

Dinner or Holiday Parties

If possible, contact your host a few days before the event and offer to bring something as an exchange you can eat. This could be a healthy, fat-filled meal that is more conducive to the keto diet while you are at the party. This will help you control the temptation of the bread and dessert courses.

Don't feel pressured into eating something that you'd rather not have. The most important thing to remember is that quality time with family and friends is important, especially when embarking on a lifestyle choice that is a long-term commitment to your health, so don't miss out. Instead, plan ahead and choose keto-friendly meals.

And if, by chance, you give into temptation, which is a reality that can occur, know that you can still get back on track. If you are on the cyclical keto diet, schedule your carb days to coincide with your time out with friends, or follow up on these cheat days with a period of intermittent fasting and exercise to get you back into ketosis.

For this reason, you may find it easier to incorporate cyclical keto or intermittent fasting into your routine, as this allows more leeway when you're out with loved ones.

Chapter 6
Fourteen-day Meal Plan

You can integrate the ketogenic diet into your lifestyle by creating your own keto meal plan, full of delicious and wholesome ingredients. This book includes a full 14-day meal plan that incorporates everything you need to start. Remember that to achieve and maintain a state of ketosis, roughly 60 to 80% of your total caloric intake needs to consist of healthy fats.

Following a meal plan will help you in several ways:

- You can save time—when you prepare meals, you can manage your time more effectively. It will eliminate last-minute shopping sprees and buying unwanted food. It cuts down what you spend on takeaway or restaurant costs. It also allows you to plan according to your set budget.
- Reduce the wastage—there is wastage in every kitchen, but you can control how much food needs to be discarded. With preparation, you only buy the ingredients you will need in the quantities you need for the cycle of your planning.
- Avoid unhealthy options—because the meals are already prepared, you will not be as tempted to eat unhealthy, last-minute options.
- Enjoy more variety—when you run on a tight schedule, you recreate the same meals, and you could be tempted to stray

from the diet. Variety will encourage you to try something new, make your meals healthier, and prevent chronic lifestyle diseases.

Whether you are an expert or just enjoy being in the kitchen with little knowledge of what you are doing, being faced with a set menu can be daunting.

The recipes mentioned are a guideline for you to kickstart your journey on keto. You can add foods that you prefer within the calorie count to make them more appealing to your taste. Each recipe can be divided into manageable portions and saved in the fridge for two to three days or in the freezer for up to six months. Once you are comfortable with the recipes, you can adjust the ingredients to accommodate you better.

Snacking is not essential, but it is a way to increase your protein, carbohydrate or fat levels on a day that your activity levels are increased. Snacks can also be supplemented with protein shakes. You can combine your daily meal plan with a snack that can increase your protein and calorie intake while keeping your carbohydrate levels low.

Fourteen-day Eating Plan

This schedule is based on the absorption of around 50 grams of carbohydrates a day. In all cases, remember your activity level, weight-loss goals, age and gender when calculating the total of calories you require.

Week 1: Monday

Breakfast: Fried Eggs With Sautéed Greens

Greens can consist of kale, cabbage, broccoli, or other leafy vegetables. Each of them have their own flavour, texture, and cooking time. Just be aware that some greens can be bitter or peppery and taste unpleasant when cooked too long.

When cooking greens, add them last after all other ingredients are cooked through, to keep them lush and green without having them turn mushy. The best method is to lay them on top of the ingredients in your pan, put the lid back on, and turn the heat down. After about 5 minutes, stir them through the rest of the ingredients and prepare to serve.

Time: 30 minutes

Makes: 1 serving

Prep Time: 15 minutes to prepare the vegetables

Cook Time: up to 5 minutes for the eggs, plus 10 minutes for the vegetables

Ingredients:

- 2 large eggs
- 3 tbsp canola seed oil
- 67 g kale—cut into long strips (sliced)
- ½ onion—sliced or cut into squares (diced)
- ½ green pepper—sliced or diced
- ½ yellow pepper—sliced or diced

- ½ red pepper—sliced or diced
- salt and pepper—it is recommended that you taste your sauce before adding the seasoning
- optional ingredients include: 50 g of mushrooms or 115 g of diced bacon
- You can swap kale for blanched (parboiled) cabbage or spinach

Directions:

1. You need to rinse your vegetables and let them drain well.
2. Cut them up as you prefer.
3. Pour ⅔ of your oil into a pan and place over medium heat for 1 minute. To test if the oil is ready, place a small piece of onion in the pan. If it sizzles, your oil is warm enough to sauté your vegetables.
4. If you add bacon, put it in the pan and cook it until it is golden brown or crispy as you prefer. Then, scoop it out of the pan with a slotted spatula and place it on a plate lined with a paper towel.
5. Place all your vegetables in the pan except the kale, stirring often to prevent them from burning.
6. When the vegetables are soft, add the kale, and place the lid on your pan for 2 minutes. Stir the kale and place the lid back on until the kale is soft. Remember that kale, cabbage, and spinach boil down when they cook, so 113 grams of raw kale can make 56 grams when cooked.
7. Taste your sauce, then add ⅛ teaspoon of salt and pepper, and stir it through. Let it cook for about a minute and taste your sauce again. Keep in mind that bacon is also salty, so add as little salt as possible until the bacon is added.
8. Add your bacon, stir it through, and remove the pan from the heat.
9. In another pan, pour the rest of your oil to heat. Remember that the stove plate will be warmed already, so the oil won't take as long to heat.
10. With gentle taps on the shells with the side of a fork, break the eggs into the pan. Sprinkle with salt and pepper. The eggs will

take between 2 and 5 minutes to cook, depending on how you prefer your eggs. For a soft yolk, wait for the white to set. Leave the egg for a minute or two longer for a harder yolk. To remove the egg, place the edge of the spatula under the egg and tip the pan slightly until the yolk rests on the utensil, then transfer to your plate.

Lunch: Portobello Bun Cheeseburgers With Avocado and Salad

Portobello mushrooms contain antioxidants that fight disease and combat inflammation, promoting excellent heart health. They are low in calories, high in fibre and vitamin B, and boost your immune system. The flat caps of the portobello mushrooms are ideal for making burger buns.

The size of the individual patty is dependent on your preferences. It will help you to save time and money in the future to individually wrap the raw patties you're not going to use, and freeze them for a future date.

Garnishes you can try include

- sliced dill pickles
- romaine lettuce
- spicy brown mustard
- mayonnaise with chilli flakes

Time: 40 minutes

Makes: 1 patty

Prep Time: 15 minutes

Cook Time: 25 minutes

Ingredients:

- 76 g ground meat—either beef, pork, or fish
- ½ tsp Worcestershire sauce
- salt and pepper
- ⅛ tsp oregano or mixed herb
- ½ tsp avocado oil
- 2 portobello mushroom caps
- 1 slice cheddar cheese
- ¼ avocado
- 1 lettuce leaf
- 75 g cherry tomatoes cut in half
- ¼ cucumber cut in cubes
- 45 g broccoli
- ½ tsp of lemon juice
- ½ tsp olive oil

Directions:

Patties:

1. Place your meat in a mixing bowl and add the Worcestershire sauce, salt, pepper, and oregano mix. Using your hands, mix till the ingredients are well combined, forming a smooth, tacky ball. If your mix is too dry, add 1 tablespoon of avocado oil. If it is too wet, add a teaspoon of flour.
2. Divide the mix into 6 golf-ball sized circles, and put them on a board or plate. Taking a ball into your hand, gently pat it with the other hand until it takes the shape of a patty. This is the ideal time to wrap the extra individual patties and place them in the freezer.

Salad:

1. Roughly shred the lettuce leaf and place it in a bowl.
2. Slice your cucumbers into rings, and roughly cut into cubes. Add them to the lettuce.

3. Cut the tomatoes in half from the top to the bottom. Using a finely serrated knife makes it easier to cut without the tomato rolling away from the knife. Place them in the bowl with your lettuce and cucumber.

4. Cut your avocado from top to bottom and remove the stone in the centre. With the flesh up and still in its skin, take your knife and cut the fruit from side to side without breaking through the skin. Then cut across the first marks till your avocado resembles a pineapple, invert the skin, and scrape the cut diamonds from the skin into your salad bowl.

5. Cut the florets of the broccoli from its stalk and add to the salad.

6. Sprinkle with salt, pepper, lemon juice, and olive oil, and mix the ingredients through. Store in the fridge to chill while you prepare the burgers.

Burgers:

1. Pour the avocado oil into a large pan, and heat it over a medium heat. Add the mushroom caps and cook for 3 minutes on one side and then turn them over and cook for another 2 minutes, then remove from the pan.

2. In the same pan, cook the patty for 4 minutes on one side, or longer, depending on how thick it is, then flip them over and cook the other side. After flipping the patty, add a slice of cheese across it, then cover the pan with a lid for 1 minute to give the cheese a chance to melt.

Assembly:

1. To make the burger, place a portobello cap upside-down on a plate. Place a cheesy burger on it, then add whichever garnish and sauce you'd like, and top with another portobello cap. Add your salad and enjoy your meal!

Dinner: Chicken With Cream Sauce and Cauliflower

This recipe allows you to freeze what you don't use for another lunch or dinner.

Time: 30 minutes

Makes: 2 servings

Prep Time: 10 minutes

Cook Time: 20 minutes depending on the size of the chicken portions

Ingredients:

- 454 g boneless chicken -diced
- salt and pepper
- ¼ tsp paprika
- 2 tbsp butter
- 2 cloves garlic -grated
- 155 ml cream of chicken soup
- 119 ml water
- 113 g chopped cauliflower or spinach

Directions:

1. Sprinkle salt, pepper, and paprika, and with your hands massage the seasoning into the chicken until it is covered all over. Set it aside and remember to wash your hands with warm, soapy water to prevent cross contamination.
2. Put a large pan on medium heat and let it get really warm, then place half of the butter in the hot pan and let it melt.
3. Place the chicken in the pan and let it fry for about 5 minutes before turning it over. Place it on a plate, cover it lightly with some tin foil to keep warm.
4. In the same pan, melt the rest of the butter, adding the garlic until it is golden brown and gives off its fragrance. Pour the canned soup and water into the pan and mix them together until the mixture starts bubbling, then turn the heat to low.

5. Return the chicken to the creamy pan with the cauliflower or spinach and cover it with a lid. Let it cook for 10 minutes, then see if the chicken is completely done by placing your knife's point through the thickest part. If the liquid runs clear, your chicken is done.
6. If you prefer your vegetables to be more crunchy, add them after you turn the heat off. This will allow them to maintain some texture but soften.
7. Serve the meal warm. Let the food cool down completely before placing in the fridge or freezer.

Week 1: Tuesday

Breakfast: Mushroom Omelette

Omelettes are great meals that are easy to prepare and very versatile. They can be made for breakfast or lunch and are perfect for those family brunches. You can use various ingredients, including bacon, ham, shredded chicken, ground meat, fish flakes, peppers, different types of mushrooms, kale, or spinach. Also remember that if you do use salted butter, decrease the amount of salt you use for seasoning.

Time: 15 minutes

Makes: 1 serving

Prep Time: 10 minutes

Cook Time: 5 minutes

Ingredients:

- 2 eggs, scrambled
- 2 tbsp almond or coconut milk
- salt and pepper
- 1 tbsp unsalted butter
- 120 g cheddar cheese, grated
- ¼ onion, diced
- 4 large mushrooms—you can use the stalks of the portobello mushrooms used for the bunless burgers

Directions:

1. Crack the eggs into a pouring jug, add the milk, salt, and pepper, and mix them with a fork or whisk.
2. Cut your onions and mushrooms.
3. Heat a pan over medium heat and let the butter melt.
4. When the pan is warmed, place the onions into it and cook them till they become transparent. Then add the mushrooms and keep stirring until they are tender.
5. Pour the eggs around the mushrooms, letting them cook till they are nearly set, then sprinkle with the cheese.
6. With a spatula, gently flip the omelette over. When it becomes golden brown, remove from the stove. With the edge of the spatula beneath the folded edge to support the omelette, slide it onto a plate.

Lunch: Zesty Chilli Lime Tuna Salad

Tuna is a very healthy protein due to its high omega-3 content and when paired with mayonnaise, it becomes the ideal keto food.

This recipe is versatile as the fish can be swapped with another type of fish or boiled egg. Add some steamed or raw vegetables to make a plate for dinner. You can also add chopped onion, black pepper, or lemon juice.

Alternatives

You can wrap the mix into a leaf of lettuce for a desk-bound lunch meal. You can stuff half an avocado for a morning snack or as part of a light dinner, or half a bell pepper to have as an open sandwich.

Time: 5 minutes

Makes: 1 serving

Prep Time: 5 minutes

Cook Time: 0 minutes

Ingredients:

- 113 g mayonnaise
- 1 tbsp lime juice
- salt and pepper
- 1 tsp chilli lime seasoning
- 1 medium stalk celery, finely chopped
- 2 tbsp finely chopped red onion
- 47 g roughly chopped lettuce
- 142 g tin of tuna

Directions:

1. Add your mayonnaise, lime juice, salt, pepper, and chilli lime seasoning to a medium-sized mixing bowl. It makes it easier when you mix the dry ingredients together before adding in the wet ingredients, to ensure that they are evenly spread through the mix
2. Add the rest of your ingredients and stir through to ensure that they are well covered by the mayonnaise mixture.

Dinner: Meatza With Stuffed Mini Peppers

This meal is made up of two items that can be used as one meal or as separate meals with a side of steamed vegetables. Both allow you to make them as spicy as you prefer.

Time: 30 minutes

Makes: 2 meatza

Prep Time: 5 minutes

Cook Time: 25 minutes

Ingredients:

Meatza:

- 454 g minced meat—beef and/or pork, or chicken
- salt and pepper
- ½ tsp mixed herbs
- ½ red onion, thinly sliced
- ¼ green pepper, diced
- 80 g black olives—you can use green as well
- 120 g cheddar cheese
- tomato & basil sauce

Peppers:

- 454 g peppers
- 454 g minced meat of your choice
- 284 g tinned tomatoes, drained
- 227 g cream cheese, softened at room temperature
- 120 g grated cheddar cheese
- 120 g grated Monterey Jack cheese
- 2 tbsp taco seasoning
- 2 tbsp hot sauce, though this is optional

Directions:

Meatza:

1. Put your oven on 180 degrees Celsius to heat up.
2. In a bowl, place your meat and seasoning and combine until a smooth ball is formed.
3. On a baking sheet, put the meat in the centre and massage it till it forms a large, thin circle.
4. Bake for 15 minutes.
5. Spread some tomato & basil sauce over the crust, then top with simple ingredients such as red onion, black olives, green peppers, and cheddar cheese. Put it back in the oven for another 10 minutes.

Peppers:

1. Keep your oven on to 180 degrees Celsius while you continue with the rest of your preparations and grease a deep oven dish.
2. You will need to cut the peppers in half, lengthwise. Use a spoon to remove the seeds.
3. Put the peppers, openside up, in the oven dish.
4. Warm a large skillet over medium heat, add a tablespoon of butter, and once it is melted, add the minced meat of your choice, letting it brown.
5. Remove the pan from the heat and turn the stove to low while you drain the excess oil from the meat into a bowl.
6. Add the tomatoes, taco seasoning, cream cheese, 60 grams cheddar cheese, 60 grams Monterey Jack cheese, and hot sauce to the pan with the browned meat.
7. Put the pan back over the low heat and stir the ingredients until everything is mixed and the cheese is melted. Remove from the heat.
8. Spoon the mixture into the halved peppers, topping it with the rest of the cheddar and Monterey Jack cheese. Bake for 10 minutes.

Week 1: Wednesday

Breakfast: Stuffed Pepper With Cheese and Egg

You can vary the ingredients by adding bacon for extra protein.

Time: 35 minutes

Makes: 1-2 servings

Prep Time: 5 minutes

Cook Time: 30 minutes

Ingredients:

- 1 large egg
- 1 large pepper—either red, yellow, or green.
- 120 g cheese, grated
- 1 tsp chives

- salt and pepper

Directions:

1. Turn your oven to 200 degrees Celsius while you continue with the rest of your preparations. Line a baking tray with parchment paper, then lightly grease with butter.
2. Place the pepper open-side up on the tray and bake for about 20 minutes.
3. Place a tablespoon of cheese in the pepper, then pour an egg over it. Lightly sprinkle with salt and pepper.
4. Add another tablespoon of cheese around the yolk, and sprinkle with chives.
5. Put it back in the oven for another 20 minutes or until the egg white is set.

Lunch: Wild rocket Salad With Hard-Boiled Eggs, Avocado, and Blue Cheese

Time: 25 minutes

Makes: 2 servings

Prep Time: 25 minutes

Cook Time: 0 minutes

Ingredients:

- 1 avocado
- 2 eggs
- 94 g wild rocket or lettuce
- 52 g cucumber
- 2 spring onions
- 18 g pine nuts
- 30 g blue cheese
- 3 tbsp olive oil

- 2 tbsp lemon juice
- 2 tsp balsamic vinegar
- ½ tbsp Dijon mustard
- 1 clove garlic, minced
- 230 g shredded turkey, chicken, or fish (optional)

Directions:

1. Place your eggs into cold water in a saucepan on high heat, and let them come to a boil for about 5-10 minutes. Then remove them from the stove and run cold water over them.
2. Place the raw pine nuts in a pan on medium heat, then gently shake the pan to keep them moving until the nuts are done. Place them aside to cool.
3. Prepare your lettuce, cucumber, and spring onions. Slice the spring onions along the length, then place them flat on your cutting board, slice them into semicircles, and mix them all in a salad bowl.
4. Slice the avocado into rough chunks, and add to the rest of the salad.
5. Tap the eggs until the shell is cracked all over, making the peeling process easier. Cut them into cubes and slide them into the salad bowl. Add your shredded turkey, crisped bacon, or flaked fish.
6. In a pouring jug, mix the oil, lemon juice, balsamic vinegar, mustard, and garlic, and mix them all together.
7. Pour the dressing over the salad. Using two dessert spoons, place them deep under the salad, and carefully scoop them from the bottom to the top, effectively tossing it.
8. Sprinkle the cheese, pine nuts, salt, and pepper over the top, then toss to incorporate.

Dinner: Seared Salmon With Spinach and Mushrooms

Time: 25 minutes

Makes: 2 servings

Prep Time: 10 minutes

Cook Time: 15 minutes

Ingredients:

- 2 tbsp olive oil
- 2 cloves garlic
- 227 g mushrooms
- 2 tomatoes
- 60 g spinach
- salt and pepper
- 1 tbsp balsamic vinegar
- 2 salmon fillets

Directions:

1. Prepare your fish by patting it gently with a paper towel to get rid of excess moisture. Sprinkle salt and pepper on both sides, and then keep it in the fridge until you are ready to cook it.
2. Slice your garlic, mushrooms, and tomatoes in the sizes you prefer.
3. Heat half of your olive oil in a pan, and once it's warm, add the garlic and mushrooms, stirring them frequently. They will shrink in size, and when this happens, add a bit of butter so that they can become crispy.
4. Add the tomatoes and allow them to become almost squishy.
5. Lastly, put your spinach in the pan and let the heat make it soft and darken in colour. Add your salt and pepper, and mix well. Dish it onto a plate and cover it with a sheet of foil.
6. With the remaining olive oil in the pan, let it become very hot. Lay your salmon fillets, skin down, in the pan. Let them sizzle for about 5 minutes without disturbing them because they'll break. Turn them onto the other side and let them cook for 5 minutes.

7. Drizzle some balsamic vinegar over the vegetables and place your salmon on top once cooked.

Week 1: Thursday

Breakfast: Full-Fat Yoghurt Topped With Keto Granola

Time: 25 minutes

Makes: 1 cup

Prep Time: 10 minutes

Cook Time: 15 minutes

Ingredients:

- 24 g almonds
- 21 g hazelnuts
- 21 g pecans
- 7 g pumpkin seeds
- 7 g sunflower seeds
- 1 tbsp sugar
- 34 g ground/milled golden flaxseed
- white of 1 large egg
- 20 g butter or coconut oil
- ⅓ tsp of vanilla essence
- 118 ml full-fat Greek yoghurt for serving

Directions:

1. Put your oven to 165 degrees Celsius while you line a large square or rectangular baking tray or two smaller trays with parchment paper.
2. In a food processor, pulse your hazelnuts, as they are the hardest nuts. If you don't have a processor, place your nuts in a plastic bag, and then you can use a rolling pin to crush them manually. Next in line to be crushed is the pecans. Make sure that they're not too fine.
3. In a bowl, add the pumpkin seeds, sunflower seeds, sugar, and the golden flaxseed and combine till they are mixed well.
4. Use two cups: one for the egg white and another for the yolk. With the back edge of a knife, gently tap the egg till it has a crack around its width. Over one cup, slowly part the shell till the white starts running out, making sure to proceed slowly to avoid the yolk from falling into that cup. Place the yolk in the other cup and refrigerate to use within a day.
5. In a glass container, melt your butter or coconut oil in the microwave oven for 30 seconds. Then let it cool but not get cold, and add your vanilla essence and whisk together.
6. Add the egg white to your nutty mixture, then add your butter or oil mixture slowly as you are mixing. You should have a mixture that is a little tacky, but coarsely textured.
7. Pour the mixture into the centre of your baking tray, and using the back of a spoon, press it down to form a base of approximately ¼ inch.
8. Bake for 15 to 18 minutes, or till the edges turn a light brown. Let it cool completely before breaking it apart, as it will become more crisp and easier to break.
9. In a bowl or seal-tight container, pour the yoghurt and add your granola. You can also add berries for a fruity variety.

Lunch: Burrito Bowl With Beef and Cauliflower Rice

This is an ideal lunch as it can be prepared the night before and makes use of items left over from other meals.

Time: 35 minutes

Makes: 2 servings

Prep Time: 15 minutes

Cook Time: 20 minutes

Ingredients:

- 227 g minced beef
- 1 ½ tbsp olive oil
- ¼ onion, finely diced
- ½ medium head of cauliflower
- 200 g canned tomatoes, drained and diced
- ½ tsp garlic powder or 2 cloves fresh garlic, minced
- ½ tsp onion powder
- ½ tsp paprika
- ¼ tsp chilli powder, optional
- ½ tsp cumin
- 60 ml beef broth
- 240 g shredded cheese
- salt and pepper
- fresh tomatoes, diced
- ¼ red pepper, diced
- ½ jalapeño pepper, sliced into rings
- ½ avocado, diced
- ¼ red onion, finely diced
- lemon or lime slices

Directions:

1. Gently rinse the cauliflower and place it in a food processor or hand blender until it's roughly chopped.

Beef:

1. Put 1 tablespoon of olive oil into a pan and let it heat up on medium heat. Add the onion, and the fresh garlic (if you're using it), and let it cook till soft.
2. Put the mince in the pan and add the salt and pepper, cooking until it becomes brown. Remove it from the heat and place in a bowl.
3. In a jug, add the onion powder, garlic powder (if you're using it), paprika, chilli, and cumin with a tablespoon of water to make a loose, smooth paste. This will prevent it from forming lumps in your pan. Pour it into the pan where you made the mince, and let it cook for a couple of minutes. Add the canned tomatoes and beef broth, letting it cook till it bubbles gently, allowing the juices to cook away. Add more salt and pepper if it is needed.
4. Stir it through the mince and sprinkle with the cheese. Close the pan and let the cheese melt for 2 to 3 minutes.

Assembly:

1. In a bowl, dish some cauliflower, and add the beef mix over the top.
2. Add the garnish of fresh tomatoes, red onion, avocado, jalepeño, red pepper, and lemon or lime slices. When packing this meal for an office lunch, it is recommended that you pack your garnish in a separate container to add after reheating the beef.

Dinner: Sesame-Crusted Tuna Steak With Creamed Spinach

Spinach cooks down and you might need to add more leaves a little at a time until it all cooks and shrivels. It can also be frozen for up to 3 months but will wilt in a few days in the fridge.

Time: 40 minutes

Serving Size: 2 servings

Prep Time: 15 minutes

Cook Time: 25 minutes

Ingredients:

- 2 tbsp butter
- ½ tbsp minced garlic—you can use a garlic crusher, or you can use the small side of your grater, or zester, to mince the garlic cloves
- 283 g pack of spinach
- 57 g cream cheese cut into 1-inch cubes
- 60g grated parmesan cheese
- 60g double cream
- salt and pepper
- 454 g tuna steak per serving
- 1 tbsp sesame seeds
- 1 tbsp almond flour
- ½ tbsp coconut oil

Directions:

1. On a plate, mix the sesame seeds, almond flour, salt, and pepper with your fingers. Lay the tuna into the mixture and press it down, making sure that it is well-coated on all sides.
2. Let your pan heat up till the coconut oil is sizzling, and lay the steaks down. Fry them on each side, about 4-8 minutes, depending on the size of the fish. Set them aside while you prepare the rest of the meal.
3. You will need to use two pots, a medium-sized pot and a smaller pot. In the bigger pot over medium heat, you will need to melt 1 ½ tablespoons of the butter and sauté the garlic for 2 minutes, till it gives off an aroma. You then need to add the spinach and cook it for 5 minutes.
4. In the other pot, also over medium heat, you need to heat the remaining butter, cream cheese, parmesan cheese, double

cream, salt, and pepper; once smooth, pour it over the spinach mix and stir through. Serve warm beside the cooked tuna steak

Some Variants With the Spinach:

Creamed Spinach Casserole

You can make a casserole by pouring the cream and spinach mix into a greased oven dish and baking it at 150 degrees Celsius for 20 minutes, watching the cheese doesn't burn. This casserole can be paired with a protein of your choice for a full meal.

Pureed Cauliflower

You can boil 226 g of cauliflower florets until you can push a fork through them without resistance (fork-tender) and then drain them using a colander. Place them into a food processor and pulse until they are chopped. If you don't own a processor, you can place them in a plastic bag and shake them.

Add Mozzarella

Adding mozzarella to your creamed spinach will make it even creamier. You would add it just before adding the spinach.

Flavouring

You can also add garlic powder, nutmeg, red peppers or flakes, or onion powder.

Week 1: Friday

Breakfast: Baked Avocado and Egg Boats

Time: 30 minutes

Makes: 2 boats

Prep Time: 10 minutes

Cook Time: 20 minutes

Ingredients:

- 1 avocado cut in half with stone removed
- 2 medium eggs
- salt and pepper

Directions:

1. Put your oven on 200 degrees Celsius. Line a baking tray with foil.
2. Scoop out 1 to 2 tablespoons of the avocado to form a vessel for the eggs.
3. If you are opting for one of the other fillings, now would be the ideal time to prepare it—crisp your bacon and cook your vegetables in the pan, then place them into the avocado vessels, half filling them.
4. Crack an egg into each well and bake for about 13 minutes for soft yolks, 15 minutes for medium yolks, and 18 minutes for hard yolks.

Additional Toppings:

- 1 strip of bacon, diced and cooked till it's crispy
- ¼ red pepper, finely chopped
- 17 g chopped spinach
- herbs for garnish

Lunch: Caesar Salad With Chicken

This salad can be eaten on its own or as a side dish, and the chicken can be omitted to make a vegetarian dish.

Time: 1 hour 30 minutes

Makes: 2 servings

Prep Time: 15 minutes

Cook Time: 15 minutes

Ingredients:

- 2 chicken breasts, skin removed
- 1 tbsp olive oil
- ½ tbsp dried oregano
- ¼ tsp salt
- 122 g plain yoghurt
- 60 ml lemon juice
- ¼ tsp Dijon mustard
- ¼ tsp garlic powder
- ¼ tsp onion powder
- salt and pepper
- 2 eggs
- ½ head lettuce
- 1 medium avocado
- 60 g parmesan cheese, shredded
- 1 tbsp chopped chives for decoration

Directions:

1. In a pouring jug, mix your olive oil, oregano, and salt, whisking till they are well mixed. Put your chicken in a plastic bag, add the mix, and seal the bag. Gently massage the mixture into the chicken and set in the fridge for an hour.
2. Mix the yoghurt, lemon juice, mustard, garlic powder, onion powder, salt, and pepper in a bowl and refrigerate until ready for use.
3. While your chicken rests outside of the fridge for about 15 minutes, heat a large pan with olive oil over a medium-high stove. Place the chicken in the pan for 6 to 8 minutes, then flip it over and leave for about 4 to 6 minutes.
4. Put your eggs on to boil while preparing your salad—cut your lettuce into large pieces and your avocado into cubes. When your eggs have cooled, peel and cut them into quarters.
5. When your chicken is done, transfer it to a plate and let it rest. Slice it to your preferred width.

6. Place the lettuce, avocado, eggs, and chicken into a bowl. Drizzle the prepared dressing over the chicken, then sprinkle with cheese and chives.

Dinner: Pork Chops With Vegetables

Time: 40 minutes

Makes: 2 servings

Prep Time: 10 minutes

Cook Time: 30 minutes

Ingredients:

- 454 g pork chops
- 3 tbsp olive oil
- ½ tbsp dried thyme
- ¼ tsp salt
- ¼ onion, sliced
- ½ red pepper
- ½ yellow pepper
- ½ green pepper
- ½ head broccoli
- ½ head cauliflower
- ¼ tsp red pepper flakes
- 45 g pitted black and green olives, optional
- 30 g grated cheese

Directions:

1. Turn your oven on to 200 degrees Celsius while you line a baking pan with parchment paper. Place the chops in the middle of the pan and drizzle with 1 tablespoon of olive oil. Sprinkle with salt and pepper. Bake for 10 minutes.
2. Prepare your vegetables by roughly slicing or dicing them to your preference. Place them in a bowl and adding the red pepper flakes, extra salt, pepper, and thyme, mix together.
3. Pack your seasoned vegetables around the chops, and place the pan back in the oven for 20 minutes, stirring at about the 10-minute mark. You should also flip your chops to ensure they are evenly cooked.
4. Dish your pork and vegetables onto a plate and sprinkle with olives and cheese.

Week 1: Saturday

Breakfast: Cauliflower Toast Topped With Cheese and Avocado

It is a filling breakfast that doesn't take much time, and will satisfy the craving for some toast. You can also use this recipe to make sandwiches for an office lunch.

Time: 30 minutes

Makes: 2 servings

Prep Time: 10 minutes

Cook Time: 20 minutes

Ingredients:

- 1 small head of cauliflower, grated
- 1 large egg
- 60 g mozzarella cheese
- ½ tsp garlic powder
- 1 avocado, cubed
- 1 tbsp fresh lime juice

- salt and pepper

Directions:

1. Switch your oven to 220 degrees Celsius while you line a baking tray with foil.
2. Place the cauliflower in a microwave-safe bowl, add a little water and cover with cling film. With a sharp knife, poke three or four holes into the wrap, then microwave the cauliflower on high for 4 minutes. When it is completely cool, spread it on a paper towel to drain.
3. Put the cauliflower back in the bowl and add the egg, cheese, garlic powder, salt, and pepper. Mix until well combined.
4. Spoon the mixture onto the baking tray in four equal portions as evenly as possible.
5. Bake for 18 to 20 minutes or until golden brown at the edges.
6. In a small bowl, use a fork to mash the avocado, salt, pepper, and lime juice together. Spread the topping onto the toast and serve.

Lunch: Bunless Salmon Burgers Topped With Broccoli Pesto

This recipe can be made in a pan, oven, or the barbecue.

Time: 20 minutes

Makes: 1-2 servings

Prep Time: 10 minutes

Cook Time: 10 minutes

Ingredients:

- 325 g boneless salmon fillets
- 1 large egg
- 30 g roughly chopped yellow onion
- salt and pepper

- 2 tbsp butter for frying
- ½ head of broccoli, cut into small pieces
- 2 tbsp butter
- 30 g grated parmesan cheese
- salt and pepper
- 3 tbsp butter that is soft but not melted
- 2 tbsp lemon juice

Directions:

Burgers:

1. Cut the fish in pieces and place it into a food processor, adding the egg, onion, salt, and pepper. Pulse until it is a coarse mixture.
2. Shape the salmon into patties.
3. Melt the 2 tablespoons of butter in a pan over medium heat and fry the burgers for about 3 to 4 minutes each side. When barbecuing, put the burgers on low heat, turning after 3 to 4 minutes or until golden brown.

Pesto:

1. Fill a pot with water and add ¼ teaspoon of salt. when it boils, add the broccoli and let it cook until it's fork-tender, then strain.
2. Put the broccoli, 2 tablespoons of butter, and cheese in a bowl. Mash them together with a potato masher until they are combined.
3. In a separate bowl, mix together 3 tablespoons of butter and the lemon juice with a hand blender or whisk, until it's light and creamy. You can season it with salt if you used unsalted butter. Coarse black pepper can enhance the flavour.
4. Serve the warmed burgers with a dollop of lemon butter and the broccoli.

Dinner: Meatballs With Courgette Noodles and Parmesan Cheese

Courgettes make ideal vegetables to manipulate into strips for noodles.

Time: 40 minutes

Makes: 2 serving

Prep Time: 15 minutes

Cook Time: 25 minutes

Ingredients:

Meatballs:

- olive or coconut oil for frying
- 340 g beef mince
- 226 g turkey or chicken mince
- 30 g grated cheese
- 1 tsp Italian seasoning
- salt and pepper
- 1 egg, beaten
- ¼ onion, finely cubed
- 1 garlic clove, minced
- 2 tbsp almond flour
- 1 tbsp fresh parsley, chopped

Zoodles:

- ½ medium onion, finely chopped
- 1 garlic clove, finely chopped
- salt and pepper
- 1 tbsp tomato paste
- 200 g tin of tomatoes, diced
- 400 g tin of crushed tomatoes
- 118 ml beef broth
- 1 tsp dried oregano
- 1 bay leaf
- ¾ tsp dried basil

- 3 medium courgettes
- chopped parsley and cheese for serving

Directions:

1. When making the meatballs, add the minced meats, cheese, Italian seasoning, salt, pepper, onion, and garlic into a bowl. Mix in the egg, almond flour, and parsley with your hand until a tacky ball is formed. Form balls in the sizes you need.
2. To cook on the stove, heat 2 tablespoons of olive oil in a pan, adding more as you cook the meatballs for 8-10 minutes, making sure they're brown on all sides. Place them on a plate lined with a paper towel.
3. Alternatively, If you choose to use the oven, set your oven to 200 degrees Celsius. In a baking tray, place a sheet of parchment paper or foil, pack the meatballs, and bake for 15-20 minutes, making sure that they are cooked through.

Sauce:

1. allow 1 tablespoon of fresh olive oil to heat up in a small pot. Add the onions and garlic, cooking until they're transparent and fragrant, then sprinkle with salt and pepper. Add the tomato paste and let it cook for about a minute, mixing in the tomatoes, broth, oregano, and bay leaf, letting it boil gently for 20 minutes or until the sauce thickens. Stir in the basil, then place the meatballs across the top, closing the pot to let it simmer until the meat is heated.

Zoodles:

1. Peel the courgettes, and with a vegetable peeler, slice them from top to bottom in narrow ribbons.
2. In a lightly oiled pan, cook the zoodles until they are almost transparent.

3. Spoon them into a bowl, and place the meatballs on them with a scoop of sauce. Garnish by sprinkling the cheese and parsley over the bowl.

Week 1: Sunday

Breakfast: Coconut Milk Chia Pudding Topped With Coconut and Walnuts

You can have this as a breakfast, pudding, or midday snack. You can also add a variety of fruit or nuts to experiment with the flavour.

Time: 5 minutes

Makes: 2 servings

Prep Time: 5 minutes (needs to set overnight)

Cook Time: 0 minutes

Ingredients:

- 236 ml coconut milk
- 22 g chia seeds
- 11 g grated coconut
- ½ tbsp fruit syrup
- ½ tsp vanilla essence
- ½ tsp coconut essence
- 20 g raspberries for garnish
- ¼ tsp cinnamon to sprinkle

Directions:

1. Add all the ingredients, except the raspberries and cinnamon, in a jug and mix until incorporated. Set in the fridge overnight.
2. Pour into a cup and top with fruit or nuts of your choice, coconut shavings, and sprinkle cinnamon over the top.

Lunch: Cobb Salad With Greens, Eggs, Avocado, Cheese, and Turkey

Time: 20 minutes

Makes: 2 servings

Prep Time: 15 minutes

Cook Time: 5 minutes

Ingredients:

- 1 large boiled egg, chopped
- 141 g shredded lettuce
- 1 small red tomato, diced
- 60 g crumbled blue cheese
- 3 slices of bacon
- ½ avocado, sliced
- 226 g turkey breast meat, cooked
- 6 tbsp Italian dressing

Directions:

1. On medium-high heat, cook the bacon until it is crispy, then lay it on a plate covered with a paper towel.
2. Place the lettuce in a large bowl, then cover with half the salad dressing and arrange on a serving platter. Place the bacon, eggs, avocado, tomato, turkey, and blue cheese over the lettuce. Drizzle with the remaining dressing and serve.

Dinner: Coconut Chicken Curry

Time: 30 minutes

Makes: 2 servings

Prep Time: 5 minutes

Cook Time: 25 minutes

Ingredients:

- 2 tbsp olive oil
- ½ onion, diced
- 454 g chicken breast cut into cubes
- 400 g can of diced tomato, drained
- 236 ml coconut cream
- 60 ml chicken broth
- 4 garlic cloves, crushed
- 1 ½ tbsp curry powder
- 1 tsp ground ginger
- 1 tsp paprika
- salt to taste

Directions:

1. In a large pot, heat a tablespoon of oil over medium heat, add the onion and cook till it's transparent and brown
2. Add your chicken and let it brown on each side for about 2-4 minutes, adding more oil if the pot is too dry.
3. Mix the rest of your ingredients, add to the pot, and stir it all together. Let it come to a boil, lower the heat and let it simmer for about 15-20 minutes till the chicken is completely cooked and the sauce has thickened

Week 2: Monday

Breakfast: Scrambled Eggs in Butter Topped With Avocado

Time: 10 minutes

Makes: 1 serving

Prep Time: 5 minutes

Cook Time: 5 minutes

Ingredients:

- 2 large eggs
- 1 tbsp butter
- salt and pepper
- 30 g grated cheddar cheese
- 37 g avocado, cubed
- ¼ tomato, cubed

Directions:

1. Whisk your eggs, salt, and pepper in a bowl while your pan heats up over medium-high heat and let your butter melt.
2. Pour your egg into the pan and spread a layer of cheese, or other filling over the top, then lower the heat to medium.
3. Leave the eggs for 30 seconds, then take your spatula and cut through the egg to separate it and form a soft curd.
4. Leave the eggs for another 15 seconds to set. Repeat until the eggs have thickened. Gently tip them onto a plate, and garnish with tomato, avocado, and chives.

You can have the scrambled eggs on their own, topped with bacon, mushrooms, or on a slice of cauliflower toast.

Lunch: Spinach Salad With Grilled Salmon

Time: 10 minutes

Makes: 1 serving

Prep Time: 10 minutes

Cook Time: 10 minutes if you need to cook your salmon

Ingredients:

- 57 g mayonnaise
- ½ tbsp avocado oil
- ¼ tbsp apple cider vinegar
- ¼ tbsp Dijon mustard
- 1 small garlic clove, minced
- ½ tbsp fresh dill
- salt and pepper
- 15 g baby spinach
- 113 g cooked salmon
- ¼ avocado, chopped or sliced
- 1 small radish, sliced
- ½ red onion, thinly sliced

Directions:

Dressing:

- In a mason jar with a tight lid, mix your mayonnaise, avocado oil, apple cider vinegar, Dijon mustard, garlic, dill, salt, and pepper by shaking the jar vigorously.

Salad:

- Arrange your spinach on a plate or in a bowl, and set your salmon on it, either whole or cut into bite-sized pieces called flakes. Arrange your avocado, radish, and onion slices around your fish.
- Drizzle the dressing over it, and refrigerate any that is left over.

Dinner: Pork Chop With Cauliflower Mash and Red Cabbage Slaw

Time: 45 minutes

Makes: 2 servings

Prep Time: 5 minutes

Cook Time: 35 minutes

Ingredients:

- 1.8 L of water
- salt
- 1 large cauliflower, cut up
- 3 tbsp cream cheese
- 1 tbsp paprika
- 1 tsp Italian seasoning
- ¼ tsp red pepper
- ¼ tsp onion powder
- ¼ tsp garlic powder
- ¼ tsp garlic salt
- ¼ tsp pepper
- 2 pork chops
- 1 tbsp olive oil
- 3 tbsp butter
- ½ tsp minced garlic
- ¼ green or red cabbage, cut into strips
- 60 ml chicken or vegetable broth
- salt and pepper

Directions:

Cauliflower Mash:

1. Add a ½ teaspoon of salt to your water to boil in a large pot. Put your cauliflower chunks into the pot and close it to cook for about 8 minutes.
2. Drain the water and let it stand until all the water drains completely as cauliflower tends to hold moisture.
3. You can use a food processor or a whisk to cream the cauliflower, adding 2 tablespoons of butter and cream cheese until it's smooth.

Cajun Spice:

1. Mix together the paprika, Italian seasoning, red pepper, onion powder, garlic powder, garlic salt, and pepper in a bowl. Leftover spice can be kept in a jar with a tight lid.

Pork Chops:

1. Generously rub the dry cajun spice onto each side of the pork chops. Heat a pan over medium heat with 1 tablespoon of olive oil until it hot.
2. Place the pork chops in the pan and sear for 3-5 minutes on each side.Transfer them onto a plate.
3. Put 1 tablespoon of butter, minced garlic, and cabbage into the pan, allowing the cabbage to cook down a bit for about 4 minutes. Add the broth and the salt and pepper, stirring frequently.
4. When the cabbage is tender, stir in 1 tablespoon of butter, and lay the chops on top. Close the pan and let it simmer gently on low heat.
5. After 10 minutes, the chops should be done completely.

Week 2: Tuesday

Breakfast: Coffee With Butter and Coconut Oil and Eggs

Keto views coffee as a favourable asset while you are on the diet, because of its antioxidant, weight loss and low-carbohydrate properties. It plays a role in keeping you alert and increases your concentration and focus.

Time: 10 minutes

Serving Size: 1 cup

Prep Time: 6 minutes

Cook Time: 4-6 minutes for the eggs plus brewing time

Ingredients:

- 237 ml freshly brewed coffee
- 2 tbsp unsalted butter
- 1 tbsp coconut oil
- 2 eggs

Directions:

1. Boil the eggs as preferred.

Coffee:

1. Brew your coffee to your preference.
2. Add the butter and coconut oil and blend them until smooth and frothy. Serve hot.

Lunch: Tuna Salad Stuffed in Tomatoes

Time: 10 minutes

Makes: 1 serving

Prep Time: 10 minutes

Cook Time: 0 minutes

Ingredients:

- 1 tbsp onion, chopped
- 1 medium tomato
- 1 tbsp mozzarella cheese
- 140 g can of tuna, drained
- 2 tbsp balsamic vinegar
- 1 tbsp fresh basil, chopped

Directions:

1. Cut the top off the tomato, approximately ¼ of an inch, and remove the inside with a spoon.
2. Mix the rest of the ingredients in a bowl. When it's all combined, dish into the tomato and enjoy.

Dinner: Teriyaki Grilled Aubergines and Brussel Sprout Salad

Time: 35 minutes

Makes: 2 servings

Prep Time: 15 minutes

Cook Time: 20 minutes

Ingredients:

- 28 ml sesame oil
- 113 ml liquid aminos or soy sauce

- 2 garlic cloves, minced
- 1 tbsp ground ginger
- 2 tbsp fruit syrup
- 2 medium aubergines
- 1 tbsp sesame seed, toasted
- 1 tbsp olive oil and additional 113 ml for dressing
- 1 tsp chilli paste
- 56 g pecans
- 28 g pumpkin seeds
- 28 g sunflower seeds
- ½ tsp cumin
- salt and pepper
- 453 g brussel sprouts
- 1 medium lemon, juice and zest

Directions:

Aubergines:

1. In a pot over a medium heat, whisk together the sesame oil, liquid aminos or soy sauce, garlic, ginger, and fruit syrup together. Stir it frequently while it thickens, then remove from the heat.
2. Cut the stems from your aubergines, and cut along the length in slices that are ⅛ of an inch thick. Brush with the sauce and place on a hot grill.
3. Brush with more sauce because it will caramelise as you sear each side.
4. Drizzle with the remaining sauce and sprinkle with the toasted sesame seeds.

Brussel Sprouts:

1. Heat a pan over a low setting and add the tablespoon of olive oil and the chilli paste. Stir in the pecans. Toss in the pumpkin and sunflower seeds, season with cumin and salt and let it cook for about 3 minutes, stirring frequently.

2. After rinsing the brussel sprouts, cut them into thin slices and put them in a bowl.
3. Combine the remaining olive oil, lemon juice, and the zest (the finely grated lemon skin)salt and pepper, and drizzle over the brussel sprouts, marinating them for 10 minutes.
4. Toss the pecans and seeds into the sprouts just before serving with the grilled aubergines.

Week 2: Wednesday

Breakfast: Cheese, Mushroom, Broccoli, and Pepper Omelette

Time: 15 minutes

Makes: 1 serving

Prep Time: 10 minutes

Cook Time: 5 minutes

Ingredients:

- 2 eggs, beaten
- 2 tbsp coconut oil
- 22 g mushrooms, cut into small cubes
- 28 g broccoli, florets cut from the stalk and loosened
- 37 g red and yellow pepper, cubed
- 55 g crisped bacon cubes
- 60 g cheese

Directions:

1. Pour the eggs into the heated oil in a pan over low heat, giving it a chance to set but not cook through.
2. Sprinkle your ingredients onto one half of the egg mixture, then gently lift the other half over and let it cook for about 2 minutes.
3. Slide the omelette onto a plate.

Lunch: Prawns With Avocado Salad

Time: 20 minutes

Makes: 2 servings

Prep Time: 15 minutes

Cook Time: 5 minutes

Ingredients:

- 225 g raw prawns, peeled and deveined
- 1 large avocado, roughly cubed
- 74 g cherry tomatoes, diced
- ½ red onion, finely cubed
- 15 g freshly chopped coriander or parsley
- 30 g crumbled feta cheese
- 30 g cubed cheddar cheese
- 2 tbsp salted butter, melted
- 1 tbsp lime juice
- 1 tbsp olive oil
- salt and pepper

Directions:

1. In a bowl, coat the prawns with the melted butter while you heat a pan over a medium-high stove. Place them in a single layer in the pan and grill until they're pink, then flip them over, making sure that the shrimp is completely pink. Allow them to cool while assembling the rest of the salad.
2. Add the rest of the ingredients to a large bowl, pour the olive oil and lime juice over it and toss lightly.
3. Mix the shrimp into the salad and add more salt and pepper if needed.

Dinner: Roasted Chicken With Asparagus and Sautéed Mushrooms

Time: 50 minutes

Makes: 2 servings

Prep Time: 15 minutes

Cook Time: 35 minutes

Ingredients:

- 1 chicken breast, sprinkled with salt and pepper
- 226 g mushrooms, cleaned and thinly sliced
- 226 g asparagus
- ½ onion, diced
- 1 garlic clove, minced
- 28 g unsalted butter
- 60 g Mozzarella cheese, grated
- 158 ml chicken stock
- 88 ml double cream
- 158 ml Madeira wine
- parsley, chopped
- 1 tbsp extra virgin olive oil
- salt and pepper

Directions:

1. Half fill a large pot with water, and add ¼ teaspoon of salt. Place on high heat and once it boils add the asparagus. Let it cook for about 2 minutes and then drain it.
2. Take a large pan, and heat the olive oil over a medium-high stove. Once it is warm, add the mushrooms, cooking them for 2 minutes.
3. Add the onion and garlic and let it cook for another 4 minutes, then dish the ingredients into a bowl.
4. Melt the butter into the pan and gently lay the chicken breasts into the warm butter for 4-5 minutes on each side. Lower the

heat and slowly add the wine. The alcohol will evaporate, and after 2 minutes, you can remove the chicken from the pan, leaving the wine sauce.

5. Turn the heat up again while pouring the stock and cream into the pan. Mix them well and let it boil. If it is too thick, add more stock. Once it's boiling, bring the heat down again, and let it simmer for 6 minutes.

6. Season with parsley and add the chicken back into the pan. Dish the mushrooms over the chicken and the asparagus along the sides of the pan. Cover with mozzarella, and let the pan simmer with its lid on over low heat for 15 minutes, until the cheese has melted.

7. You can also place your open pan in the oven at 200 degrees Celsius for about 20 minutes.

8. Remove from the heat and serve.

Week 2: Thursday

Breakfast: Almond Milk Smoothie With Cinnamon

Time: 5 minutes

Makes: 1 serving

Prep Time: 5 minutes

Cook Time: 0 minutes

Ingredients:

- 118 ml coconut milk
- 118 ml unsweetened almond milk or water
- 1 tbsp coconut oil or MCT oil
- ½ tsp ground cinnamon
- 1 tbsp chia seeds
- 30 g vanilla or plain whey protein powder
- ice

Directions:

1. Combine the coconut milk, protein powder, cinnamon, and chia seeds in a blender.
2. Add the coconut or MCT oil, almond milk or water, and ice. Blend until it's smooth, pour it into a glass garnished with cinnamon, and serve.

Lunch: Chicken With Cucumber and Goat's Cheese

Time: 30 minutes

Makes: 1 serving

Prep Time: 10 minutes

Cook Time: 20 minutes

Ingredients:

- 60 g spinach leaves
- 1 small cucumber, cubed
- 1 avocado, cubed
- 50 g goat's cheese or feta, cubed
- juice of ½ lime
- 59 ml sour cream
- 1 tbsp chopped chives
- salt and pepper
- 3 tbsp almond flour
- 3 tbsp grated parmesan cheese
- ¼ tsp dried basil and thyme mixed
- 113 g chicken breast, cut into strips
- 2 tbsp butter

Directions:

Salad:

1. Using either whole or chopped spinach leaves, place them in a bowl. Spread your cucumber and avocado chunks over the top.
2. Gently rub the goat's cheese or feta between your fingers to crumble them.
3. Pour the lime juice over, as well as the sour cream and chives. Sprinkle with salt and pepper, and toss to mix them together.

Chicken

1. Turn your oven on to 190 degrees Celsius, then line a baking tray with foil.
2. In a bowl, combine your almond flour, parmesan cheese, basil and thyme mix, salt, and pepper.
3. In a separate bowl, melt your butter. Don't let it get too hot, you should be able to dip your finger in without burning.
4. Place your chicken pieces into the butter then coat them in the dry ingredient mixture and place them on the baking tray.
5. Bake for 20 minutes until the chicken's juices run clear when poked, and the chicken is golden brown on the outside.
6. Place the cooked strips on the tossed salad, and enjoy.

Dinner: Grilled Lemon Butter Prawn With Asparagus

Time: 25 minutes

Makes: 1 serving

Prep Time: 10 minutes

Cook Time: 15 minutes

Ingredients:

- 133 g prawns, peeled and deveined
- ¼ tbsp grated ginger
- ¼ tbsp chopped leek
- 1 garlic clove, chopped
- ½ tsp lemon juice
- ½ tsp soy sauce or coconut aminos
- 1 tbsp butter
- salt and pepper
- 166 g asparagus

Directions:

1. Put your oven on at 180 degrees Celsius.
2. Cut the bottom of the stems of your asparagus and rinse thoroughly. You can then boil them in a pot of water for 2 minutes with a ½ teaspoon of salt, and then strain.
3. Melt the butter, add soy sauce or coconut aminos in a bowl, and stir until well-blended.
4. Marinade the prawns with the ginger, garlic, lemon juice, leek, salt, and pepper.
5. In a baking tray lined with foil and rubbed with oil, arrange the asparagus in one part of the tray, with the shrimp in the other. Drizzle the remaining sauce over.
6. Bake until the prawns turns pink, approximately 10-15 minutes. Remove from the oven and serve.

Week 2: Friday

Breakfast: Mushrooms Stuffed With Sausage and Cheese

Time: 40 minutes

Makes: 8-16 mushrooms

Prep Time: 15 minutes

Cook Time: 25 minutes

Ingredients:

- 227 g sausage, skinned
- 60 g cream cheese
- 60 g grated cheddar cheese
- 450 g large mushrooms, stems removed and halved
- salt and pepper
- chopped chives, optional

Directions:

1. Put your oven on 200 degrees Celsius.
2. Cook the sausage meat over medium heat.
3. After draining the fat, add all the cheeses—keeping 30 g of cheddar aside—salt, and pepper and stir.
4. Spoon the cheese and meat mixture into the mushrooms and sprinkle with the rest of the cheese. Bake for 25 minutes. Sprinkle the chives before serving.

Lunch: Burgers in Lettuce Topped With Avocado, and Salad

Time: 20 minutes

Makes: 2 servings

Prep Time: 10 minutes

Cook Time: 10 minutes

Ingredients:

- ¼ large head of lettuce
- 283 g beef mince
- ¼ tsp of Cajun spice
- 1 medium tomato
- 1 medium onion
- 1 slice of cheddar cheese per patty

- ¾ tbsp plain Greek yoghurt
- ¼ tbsp vinegar or lemon juice
- salt and pepper
- ¾ tbsp light sour cream
- ½ tsp fruit syrup
- ½ avocado

Directions:

1. Rinse your vegetables and dry with a paper towel.
2. Slice your onions and tomato in rounds.

Burger:

1. Put your mince, Cajun spice, and salt into a bowl and combine. Divide roughly into eight balls and shape them into patties. This would be the time to freeze any patties you don't use.
2. Add a tablespoon of olive oil to a heated pan and place the patties in it. Cook for about 5 minutes per side, depending on the thickness of the patty, until there is no pink juice running from the centre. Place a slice of cheese on each patty after you've flipped it.

Sauce:

1. Mix the yoghurt, vinegar or lemon juice, salt, pepper, sour cream, and fruit syrup really well in a bowl or bottle.

Assembly:

1. Lay two lettuce leaves on your board, place a slice of tomato and onion slightly towards the top, and put some sauce on it. If you prefer, you may fry your onions before adding it to the lettuce
2. Add the burger and top with slices of avocado.

3. Fold the bottom edge of the lettuce over the stack and fold the sides in, forming a vessel.

Dinner: Beef Stew With Mushrooms, Onions, Celery, and Herbs

The remaining food can be divided into ideal portions, frozen, and easily reheated.

Time: 1 hour 45 minutes

Makes: 2 servings

Prep Time: 15 minutes

Cook Time: 1 hour 30 minutes

Ingredients:

- 227 g beef roast, cut into pieces
- salt and pepper
- 1 tbsp olive oil
- 113 g mushrooms, sliced
- ½ chopped onion
- 1 small carrot, cut into discs
- 1 stalk celery, sliced
- 1 garlic clove, minced
- ½ tbsp tomato paste
- 711 ml beef broth
- ½ tsp fresh thyme leaves
- ½ tsp freshly chopped rosemary

Directions:

1. On medium heat, put oil into a large pot and let it warm, then sear your beef for about 3-5 minutes per side. Put on a plate.
2. Place the mushrooms in the pot and let them cook till golden, then cook the onions, carrot, and celery until they are soft. Add the garlic, and sauté for about 1 minute, then stir in the tomato paste.
3. Put the beef back in the pot with the broth, thyme, and rosemary, and season with salt and pepper. Reduce to low heat and let it simmer for about 50 minutes to an hour, stirring occasionally, until you are able to cut the beef with a wooden spoon.

Week 2: Saturday

Breakfast: Keto Breakfast Pancakes

Time: 30 minutes

Makes: 5 pancakes, depending on the size of the ladle

Prep Time: 5 minutes

Cook Time: 2-3 minutes per pancake

Ingredients:

- 17 g almond flour
- 57 g cream cheese
- 2 large eggs
- ½ tsp lemon zest or vanilla essence
- ½ tbsp cocoa
- butter to fry with

Alternate toppings:

- parmesan or cheddar cheese
- unsweetened roasted coconut

- warm unsweetened peanut butter
- handful of berries
- sprinkling of bacon
- chocolate chips

Directions:

1. Pour the almond flour into a mixing bowl, making a 'well' in the centre for your cream cheese and eggs. Add the lemon zest or vanilla, and gently whisk the ingredients together until they form a smooth batter.
2. Warm a pan over medium-low heat, then add 1 tablespoon of butter to melt.
3. Using a small soup ladle, spoon 1 ladle of batter into the pan. Let it cook for 2 minutes or until it's golden, then flip it with a spatula, and let the other side cook in the same way. Transfer it to a plate and add the topping of your choice, while cooking the rest of the batter.
4. If the pan becomes dry in the cooking process, add another tablespoon of butter.
5. For a chocolate pancake, add ½ tablespoon of cocoa powder to the flour and mix it with your dry ingredients.

To soften your cream cheese, take it out of the fridge and let it stand at room temperature for at least an hour before using.

Lunch: Poached Salmon Avocado Rolls Wrapped in Seaweed

This meal makes for the ideal lunchbox. You can also swap the seaweed for kale.

Time: 15 minutes

Makes: 2 servings

Prep Time: 15 minutes

Cook Time: 0 minutes

Ingredients:

- smoked salmon, sliced into thin ribbons
- 3 small cucumbers, cut to matchstick-size
- ½ onion or leeks cut into long strips
- 1 avocado, thinly sliced
- 2 full nori seaweed sheets, or kale leaves
- 1 tsp sesame oil
- soy sauce or gluten-free wasabi

Directions:

1. Cut your ingredients according to the size of your kale leaves/seaweed sheet, so that they are just sticking out of it.
2. Layer your salmon strip, avocado, cucumber, and onion or leek on the top of the seaweed sheet or kale. Roll the sheet tightly around the filling and liberally use oil to seal it. You can use a toothpick to keep it closed.
3. Repeat the process until all the seaweed or kale leaves is used. Cut each roll into the preferred size.
4. Dip into soy sauce and wasabi, or your favourite salad dressing.

Dinner: Grilled Beef Kebabs With Peppers

This recipe allows you to add any combination of meat or fish with vegetables of your choice. You can also make it a vegetarian or vegan meal by omitting the meat completely. For a breakfast twist, add 2 boiled eggs to the skewer.

Time: 50 minutes

Makes: 2 skewers

Prep Time: 40 minutes

Cook Time: 10 minutes

Ingredients:

- 340 g sirloin steak, cut into 1-inch cubes
- ½ small red onion
- 1 pepper cubed
- ½ tsp salt
- ½ tbsp olive oil
- 30 ml soy sauce
- 30 ml balsamic vinegar
- 1 tbsp Worcestershire sauce
- ½ tsp garlic powder
- ½ tsp of Italian seasoning

Directions:

Marinade:

1. Prepare the marinade by placing your cubed steak, soy sauce, balsamic vinegar, Worcestershire sauce, garlic powder, Italian seasoning and salt in a sealed bag and massage until the meat is covered, then leave it in the fridge for about 30 minutes.
2. Soak your skewers if you are using wood skewers.
3. Cut your vegetables into about 1-inch cubes.
4. Heat your grill to 200 degrees Celsius while you assemble your kebabs.

Assembly:

1. Alternate your steak, onion, and pepper cubes onto your skewers, then brush with olive oil and salt.
2. Grill the kebabs for approximately 4-5 minutes a side, depending on how you like your steak, brushing with the remainder of the marinade.

Week 2: Sunday

Breakfast: Egg Muffins With Cheddar Cheese, Spinach, and Tomato

These muffins are very versatile because of the numerous combinations that can be created with different ingredients.

Time: 30 minutes

Makes: 3 muffins

Prep Time: 10 minutes

Cook Time: 25 minutes

Ingredients:

- 2 eggs
- ¼ red onion, chopped
- 40 g chopped spinach
- ¼ chopped green pepper
- 1 tbsp chopped mushrooms
- 40 g grated cheese
- ⅛ tsp turmeric
- salt and pepper

Suggested ingredients:

- kale
- chopped jalapeño pepper
- roasted garlic
- chopped courgettes

Directions:

1. Put your oven on 180 degrees Celsius and grease a muffin pan with coconut oil.
2. To make pouring the ingredients into the muffin tins easier, whisk your eggs in a mixing jug. Add your salt and pepper to taste. Add the other ingredients and stir them well.
3. Gently pour the mix into your muffin pan, filling the cups about two-thirds so as to avoid the mixture cooking over. Bake them for about 20-25 minutes or until the eggs have a golden-

brown colour. Depending on the size of your muffin cups, you should get about three or four muffins.

4. Allow them to cool, and enjoy with keto coffee, or add a salad to the muffins for lunch.

Lunch: Spiced Cauliflower Soup With Bacon Pieces

Time: 30 minutes

Makes 3 servings

Prep Time: 5 minutes

Cook Time: 25 minutes

Ingredients:

- ¼ cauliflower cut into large chunks
- 2 bacon strips
- ½ tsp olive oil
- 136 ml coconut milk
- 158 ml broth or water
- ¼ onion, cut into cubes
- 1 garlic clove, minced
- ½ tsp coconut aminos or soy sauce
- ¼ tsp paprika
- ¼ tsp cayenne pepper
- salt and pepper
- ¼ tsp cumin
- coriander for garnish

Directions:

1. In a large pot, cook your onions and garlic with the olive oil till they are transparent. Add the cauliflower, broth, coconut milk, paprika, cayenne pepper, salt, pepper, coconut aminos or soy sauce, and cumin. Let cook for about 10-15 minutes.

2. In the meantime, fry the bacon in a pan on medium heat, then cut into pieces and put aside.
3. When the cauliflower is tender, use an immersion blender and purée the soup.
4. Ladle into a bowl, add the bacon, and decorate with sprigs of coriander.

Dinner: Broiled Trout With Butter and Sautéed Pak Choi

Time: 25 minutes

Makes: 1 serving

Prep Time: 10 minutes

Cook Time: 15 minutes

Ingredients:

- ½ tbsp honey or fruit syrup
- 1 tbsp tamari or soy sauce
- 1 large minced garlic clove
- ¾ tsp chilli powder
- 170 g fillet of trout fish, skin on
- salt and pepper
- 2 heads of pak choi, or you can use broccoli
- ½ tsp sesame oil
- ¼ tsp pepper flakes

Directions:

1. Set your oven to 220 degrees Celsius, and line a baking tray with parchment paper.
2. Mix the honey or fruit syrup, minced garlic, chilli powder, and half of the tamari or soy sauce in a bowl.
3. Put the fish, skin down, on the parchment paper, and sprinkle with salt and pepper. You can use a pastry brush to coat the fish with the garlic mixture.
4. In a bowl, drizzle the Pak choi or broccoli with the leftover tamari or soy sauce and sesame oil, and coat liberally. Pack it around the fish.
5. Bake for 12-15 minutes or until the fish is flaky.

Snack 1: Guacamole

This is a fantastic addition to a grilled protein like fish or meat. It is ideal for the ketogenic diet and provides great fibre while keeping the carbohydrate content low.

To dip, you can use keto-friendly alternatives such as, low-carbohydrate crackers, cucumbers, or stuffed mini peppers.

Time: 15 minutes

Makes: 1 serving

Prep Time: 15 minutes

Cook Time: 0 minutes

Ingredients:

- 1 avocado, sliced and stone removed
- ½ tbsp sour cream
- ¼ diced tomatoes
- ¼ diced red onion
- 1 small garlic clove
- ¼ jalapeño pepper
- 20 g coriander
- ¼ lime
- ⅛ tsp cumin
- salt

Directions:

1. Scoop the avocado into a mixing bowl and mash it with a fork until it is the texture that you would like.
2. Stir in the sour cream.
3. Add the tomato and onion.
4. You will need to mince the garlic clove, jalapeño pepper, and coriander and add it to the avocado mix.
5. Roll a lime on the counter to loosen the fibres so that it will release the juice easier. Cut it into quarters and squeeze one

into your mixture.

6. Sprinkle your salt and cumin into the mixture and mix it well, still using a fork to keep the mixture loose.

7. Taste the mixture, and add any ingredient that you feel needs to be increased.

Snack 2: Beef Roll Ups

Time: 30 minutes

Makes: 1-2 roll ups

Prep Time: 10 minutes

Cook Time: 20 minutes

Ingredients:

- ¼ pepper, thinly sliced
- ¼ red onion, thinly sliced
- 1 slice of roast beef
- 22 g cheddar cheese, grated
- ½ teaspoon avocado or olive oil

Directions:

1. Set your oven to 180 degrees Celsius while you line a baking sheet with parchment paper.

2. Toss your pepper and onion with ½ teaspoon of avocado or olive oil in a warm pan until it's soft, then set aside.

3. Lay the beef on the baking tray in a single layer and spread the cheese across it. Place in the oven for 5 minutes or until the cheese melts. Allow to cool but not get cold.

4. Put a spoonful of vegetables at one end of the beef and roll. You can choose to slice them in half.

Snack 3: Kale Crisps

Time: 20 minutes

Makes: 2 servings

Prep Time: 10 minutes

Cook Time: 10 minutes

Ingredients:

- ½ bunch of kale
- ½ tbsp olive oil
- ½ tsp salt

Directions:

1. Preheat your oven to 175 degrees Celsius, and line a baking tray with parchment paper.
2. Cut the leaves from the stems of the kale, rinse and dry thoroughly before drizzling with olive oil and salt.
3. Bake for about 10-15 minutes, until the edges are brown.

Snack 4: Stuffed Jalapeno Fat Bombs

Time: 25 minutes

Makes: 2 halves

Prep Time: 10 minutes

Cook Time: 15 minutes

Ingredients:

- 1 jalapeño pepper, cut along the length and remove seeds
- 22 g lean beef mince
- 17 g cream cheese
- 20 g cheddar cheese, grated

- ½ slice cooked bacon
- 4 g pork scratchings (optional)

Directions:

1. Set your oven to 250 degrees Celsius and line a baking tray with foil.
2. In a mixing bowl, mix the cream cheese and cheddar cheese until soft and creamy.
3. Over medium heat, cook the beef for about 5 minutes or until brown.
4. In the open pepper, spoon some beef and cover with the cheese mix. Arrange on the baking sheet and bake for 10 minutes.
5. Cut up the pork scratching and the bacon until fine, and sprinkle onto the baked peppers. Serve while warm.

Snack 5: Pizza Cups

Time: 30 minutes

Makes: 2 servings

Prep Time: 10 minutes

Cook Time: 20 minutes

Ingredients:

- 28 g cream cheese
- 180 g grated mozzarella cheese
- 1 egg, beaten
- 136 g almond flour
- 2 tbsp coconut flour
- 75 g tomato sauce
- 40 g of cheddar cheese
- 17 g mini pepperoni slices

Directions:

1. Preheat your oven to 200 degrees Celsius, and grease a muffin tray.
2. Combine the cream cheese and mozzarella in a microwave-safe bowl, and heat for 1 minute, stirring frequently. Stir in the egg until the mixture forms a small ball. Knead in the flours until a tacky ball is formed.
3. Make eight balls from the dough, and roll each of them out, pressing each into a cup of the muffin tray. Bake them for 15 minutes.
4. Once you take them out of the oven, add the sauce, cheddar cheese, and pepperoni. Bake for a further 5 minutes.
5. Remove from the pan and serve.

Snack 6: Chocolate Fat Bombs

Time: 1 hour

Makes: 5 fat bombs

Prep Time: 1 hour

Cook Time: 0 minutes

Ingredients:

- 1 tbsp butter
- 20 g peanut butter
- ¼ tsp vanilla essence
- 2 g sugar or sugar replacement
- 28 g peanut powder
- 28 g semi-sweet chocolate chips
- ¼ tbsp MCT oil

Directions:

1. Place some parchment paper in a baking tray that is freezer-friendly.
2. Microwave the butter for 10 seconds at a time until most of it is melted. Stir in the peanut butter and microwave for another 20 seconds. The mix should be smooth and runny.
3. Combine with your vanilla, sugar or sugar replacement, and peanut powder until it forms a stiff dough.
4. With two teaspoons, scoop a portion and roll into a ball with your hands. Set it to freeze for 20 minutes or longer.
5. In the microwave, melt the chocolate chips for 20 seconds, stirring occasionally until it's melted. Stir in the MCT oil and stir until smooth.
6. Take your frozen dough balls, roll between your hands again and freeze for another 20 minutes.
7. Using a toothpick, dip each ball into your chocolate and cover, then place back on the tray. Freeze for another 5-10 minutes and store in a sealed container in the fridge.

Snack 7: Cheese and Ranch Pinchos

Time: 1 hour 30 minutes

Makes: 4 pinchos

Prep Time: 1 hour 30 minutes

Cook Time: 0 minutes

Ingredients:

- 56 g cream cheese
- ¼ tbsp mayonnaise
- ½ tbsp sour cream
- 30 g cheddar cheese
- 7 g ranch seasoning

- 1 slice of bacon, cooked and chopped
- 15 g pecans, finely chopped
- ½ tbsp chives, minced

Directions:

1. Combine your cream cheese, mayonnaise, sour cream, cheese, and ranch seasoning until fully incorporated. Chill for 1 hour.
2. When the cheese mixture is chilled, scoop small portions into your hand, roll into balls and place on a baking sheet lined with parchment paper.
3. Cover each ball by rolling it in the bacon, pecans, and chives, then refrigerate for another 30 minutes before serving.

Snack 8: Chocolate Peanut Butter Bombs

Time: 1 hour 10 minutes

Makes: 4 bombs

Prep Time: 1 hour 10 minutes

Cook Time: 0 minutes

Ingredients:

- 32 g peanut butter
- 1 tbsp coconut oil
- 4 g cocoa powder
- ¼ tsp liquid stevia
- pinch of salt, not required if the peanut butter is salted

Directions:

1. Use cupcake liners to line a small muffin tray.

2. Into a large pouring jug, add the peanut butter and the coconut oil, and microwave for 15 seconds at a time, stirring frequently until the oil is melted.
3. Add the remaining ingredients and stir until the batter is combined and smooth. Pour the batter until the muffin cups are ¾ filled, filling about 4 cups.
4. After freezing for about an hour, store them in an airtight container in the freezer. They soften quickly once removed from the freezer.

Snack 9: Pistachio and Chocolate Balls

Time: 30 minutes

Makes: 5 balls

Prep Time: 15 minutes and 15 minutes freeze time

Cook Time: 0 minutes

Ingredients:

- 42 g pistachios, shelled
- 16 g chocolate, finely chopped
- 6 g coconut flour or protein powder
- 10 g cocoa powder
- 25 g almond butter
- ¼ tsp of maple syrup
- ¼ tsp of vanilla essence
- extra ground pistachio or cocoa powder to coat

Directions:

1. Blend or manually crush the pistachios till fine, then add it to the other dry ingredients. Mix in the almond butter, syrup and the vanilla essence.
2. Knead through the ingredients with your hands.

3. Roll into bite-sized balls and place on a lined baking sheet.
4. Freeze for about an hour. Roll the frozen balls in the ground pistachio or cocoa powder.
5. Keep frozen or refrigerated.

Snack 10: Coffee Chocolate Bark Candy

Time: 15 minutes

Makes: 113 g of chocolate

Prep Time: 15 minutes

Cook Time: 0 minutes

Ingredients:

- 14 g coconut oil
- 56 g dark chocolate
- 42 g milk chocolate
- 2-3 g ground coffee

Directions:

1. Line a baking sheet with parchment paper.
2. In a glass bowl, mix the coconut oil and dark chocolate, microwaving at 30-second intervals, constantly stirring, until the chocolate is melted.
3. Add the milk chocolate and microwave for 20 seconds or until the chocolate is fully melted.
4. Combine the ground coffee into the chocolate and pour into the baking sheet, spreading with a spoon.
5. Place in the fridge/freezer until the chocolate has hardened. Break into pieces and serve.

More snack suggestions:

- almond and cheddar cheese cups
- half an avocado stuffed with chicken salad
- trail mix with unsweetened coconut, nuts and seeds
- one hard-boiled egg
- coconut chips
- olives and sliced salami
- celery with peppers and cream cheese
- berries with heavy whipped cream
- sunflower seeds
- celery and pepper strips dipped in guacamole
- macadamia nuts
- plain yoghurt topped with crushed pecans
- sliced cheese and bell pepper slices
- 20 grams of walnuts with 20 grams of berries
- celery sticks dipped in almond butter
- dried seaweed strips and cheese

Afterword

The one thing we have found in this book is that the ketogenic diet is not just a cry for attention or a passing fad but a commitment to a healthy lifestyle. And as with anything that affects your physical health, whether negatively or positively, consult with your doctor before trying it, especially if you have a chronic illness.

There is a wealth of information that speaks for or against the diet, but what is evident is that there are a number of short-term and long-term health benefits that can be enjoyed if consistency is maintained. Some people struggle to adjust to the schedule and calculations needed for the diet; however, the most important thing that needs to be remembered is the fat to carbohydrate ratio. There is a wealth of nutrition apps and meal service providers that can help make this process simpler, and once you have found your balance, keto is a pleasure to be on.

The keto flu and keto breath are potential downsides of the diet that occur as your body adapts to using fats as its new energy source. This is a temporary state that should last a few weeks and is managed mostly by drinking more water to flush the adverse minerals from your body and eating various nutrient-dense foods.

The basic rule of keto is that you need to restrict your carbohydrate intake. This doesn't mean you must eliminate carbohydrates completely from your diet, as they are essential for certain brain and body functions. The principle is that the majority of carbohydrates consumed on the diet should be non-starchy and high in dietary fibre instead of carbohydrates like white bread, rice and pasta.

Once you've reached ketosis and start using fat as your main energy source, you could become more energised and less hungry and see your risk rate for a number of health conditions reduce significantly. You could also experience a significant weight loss and by increasing your protein levels, you can build muscle mass too.

By preparing a meal plan, tracking your macronutrients, and documenting your progress, you will understand what makes you feel good and learn how your body responds to certain levels of carbohydrates, fats, and proteins. Many foods adhere to the keto diet and the diet itself can be easily adapted. For example, it can be adjusted for people who prefer vegetarian, vegan or pescatarian meals and even those who lead highly active lifestyles.

As with any eating plan, if you are not participating in a training regime, you need to burn more calories than you take in. Otherwise, you may struggle to achieve your weight loss goals. Remember to adjust your carbohydrate intake in accordance to the activity you plan on doing. Adjusting your carbohydrates for high-intensity workout days will ensure that you maintain muscle mass and have a sure supply of energy for short, strong spells of physical activity.

Keto is a low-carbohydrate, medium-protein and high-fat eating plan with many benefits to your health, especially to your heart and brain. With dedication, perseverance, patience and commitment, you can maintain the keto diet of your choice, whether it is the traditional version or the more relaxed version that allows you to just monitor your carbohydrate count and have a night out with friends. Whichever you choose, you are on track to living a healthy lifestyle and maintaining your dream body.

Bibliography

Abrams, V. (2020, May 8). *Keto pan seared salmon with sauteed mushrooms & spinach recipe.* Tasteaholics. https://www.tasteaholics.com/recipes/pan-seared-salmon-with-sauteed-mushrooms-spinach/

Adams, A. (n.d.). *Creamy chicken, bacon and cauliflower bake.* Taste.com.au. https://www.taste.com.au/recipes/creamy-chicken-bacon-cauliflower-bake-recipe/k5cbt2ej?r=healthy/x9a0fld8

Ajaeroh, N. (2021, July 29). The best low-carb cheeseburger lettuce wraps. *Nkechi Ajaeroh.* https://nkechiajaeroh.com/kechis-kitchen/low-carb/the-best-low-carb-cheeseburger-lettuce-wraps/

Amir, S. (n.d.). The best 7 anti-inflammatory foods on a ketogenic diet. *Perfect Keto.* https://perfectketo.com/anti-inflammatory-foods/

Annie. (n.d.). *Cajun pork chops with fried cabbage (Keto + one pan).* The Best Keto Recipes. https://thebestketorecipes.com/cajun-pork-chops-with-fried-cabbage-keto-one-pan/

Aobadia, A. (n.d.-a). *Keto fried chicken with broccoli and butter.* Diet Doctor. https://www.dietdoctor.com/recipes/keto-fried-chicken-broccoli-butter/servings/2

Aobadia, A. (n.d.-b). *Keto salmon burgers with mash & lemon butter.* Diet Doctor. https://www.dietdoctor.com/recipes/keto-salmon-burgers-mash-lemon-butter

Appel, L. J., Sacks, F. M., Carey, V. J., Obarzanek, E., Swain, J. F., Miller, E. R., Conlin, P. R., Erlinger, T. P., Rosner, B. A., Laranjo, N. M., Charleston, J., McCarron, P., Bishop, L. M. (2005). Effects of protein, monounsaturated fat, and carbohydrate intake on blood pressure and serum lipids: results of the OmniHeart randomized trial. *JAMA, 294*(19), 2455–2464. https://doi.org/10.1001/jama.294.19.2455

Arnarson, A. (2019, July 29). *Antioxidants explained in simple terms.* Healthline. https://www.healthline.com/nutrition/antioxidants-explained

Atkins (n.d). *Keto turkey cobb salad recipe.* https://www.atkins.com/recipes/turkey-cobb-salad/154

Azure, T. (2017, June 27). *Herb butter salmon and asparagus foil packs.* Creme de La Crumb. https://www.lecremedelacrumb.com/herb-butter-salmon-asparagus-foil-packs/#wprm-recipe-container-19812

Bansal, D. G. (2017, September 22). *How ketogenic diets curb inflammation in the brain.* UC San Francisco. https://www.ucsf.edu/news/2017/09/408366/how-ketogenic-diets-curb-inflammation-brain

Barañano, K. W., & Hartman, A. L. (2008). The ketogenic diet: Uses in epilepsy and other neurologic illnesses. *Current Treatment Options in Neurology, 10*(6), 410–419. https://doi.org/10.1007/s11940-008-0043-8

Biegel, K. L. (n.d.). *Chicken cauliflower "fried rice."* Food Network. https://www.foodnetwork.com/recipes/katie-lee/chicken-cauliflower-fried-rice-3588745#/

Bradley, S., & Mahtani, N. (2020, November 24). 25 Vegetarian keto recipes that make it totally possible to stay plant-based on the diet. *Women's Health.* https://www.womenshealthmag.com/weight-loss/g28942069/vegetarian-keto-recipes/

Bree. (2021, July 22). *Sausage and cheese keto stuffed mushrooms*. Keto Pots. https://ketopots.com/keto-stuffed-mushrooms

Buenfeld, S. (n.d.). *Mexican egg roll*. BBC Good Food. https://www.bbcgoodfood.com/recipes/mexican-egg-roll

Burke, L. M. (2020). Ketogenic low CHO, high-fat diet: The future of elite endurance sport? *The Journal of Physiology, 599*(3), 819-843. https://doi.org/10.1113/jp278928

Cabeca, A. (2019, October 24). *Why the ketogenic diet is great for hormone balance*. Mindbodygreen. https://www.mindbodygreen.com/articles/why-the-ketogenic-diet-is-great-for-hormone-balance

Campbell, K. (2020a, April 28). *Keto guacamole*. That Low Carb Life. https://thatlowcarblife.com/keto-guacamole/

Campbell, K. (2020b, June 5). *Taco stuffed mini peppers*. That Low Carb Life. https://thatlowcarblife.com/taco-stuffed-mini-peppers/

Campos, M. (2018, October 18). What is keto flu? *Harvard Health Blog*. https://www.health.harvard.edu/blog/what-is-keto-flu-2018101815052

Carb Manager. (n.d.). *Keto bacon, chicken and cheese salad*. https://www.carbmanager.com/recipe-detail/ug:fdf1d68e-8f34-eff9-78a9-865a44c9e911/keto-bacon-chicken-and-cheese-salad

Chatterjee, S. (2018, May 26). *Tuna salad stuffed tomatoes - low carb/keto lunch*. Tasty Fitness Recipes. https://www.tastyfitnessrecipes.com/tuna-salad-stuffed-tomatoes/

Cherrier, C. (2021a, January 31). *Easy shrimp avocado salad with tomatoes*. Eatwell101. https://www.eatwell101.com/shrimp-avocado-salad-recipe

Cherrier, C. (2021b, July 30). *Keto burrito bowl with beef and cauliflower rice*. Eatwell101. https://www.eatwell101.com/keto-burrito-bowl-recipe

Ciccarelli, L. (n.d.). The 7-day keto meal plan for weight loss. *Perfect Keto*. https://perfectketo.com/keto-weight-loss-meal-plan/

Claudepierre, C. (2021a, September 1). *Keto blueberry pancakes - cream cheese pancakes*. Sweet As Honey. https://www.sweetashoney.co/keto-blueberry-pancakes-cream-cheese-pancakes

Claudepierre, C. (2021b, November 26). *Keto scrambled eggs with avocado - 1.5 g net carbs*. Sweet As Honey. https://www.sweetashoney.co/keto-scrambled-eggs/

Claudepierre, C. (2021, December 14). *Keto peanut butter smoothie - best keto smoothie - dairy-free*. Sweet As Honey. https://www.sweetashoney.co/keto-peanut-butter-smoothie/

Cleveland Clinic. (n.d.). *Ketogenic diet (keto diet) for epilepsy*. https://my.clevelandclinic.org/health/treatments/7156 ketogenic diet keto diet for epilepsy

Cole2585. (n.d.). *Grain-free chicken tenders*. Allrecipes. https://www.allrecipes.com/recipe/230876/grain-free-chicken-tenders/

Coleby, A. (2021, June 7). *Rainbow veggie skewers*. Keto & Low Carb Vegetarian Recipes. https://ketovegetarianrecipes.com/rainbow-veggie-skewers-low-carb/

Cooking Point. (2020, June 27). *Cheesy broccoli meatza*. https://cookingpoint.net/cheesy-broccoli-meatza/

Craig, C. (2015). Mitoprotective dietary approaches for myalgic encephalomyelitis/chronic fatigue syndrome: Caloric restriction, fasting, and ketogenic diets. *Medical Hypotheses, 85*(5), 690–693. https://doi.org/10.1016/j.mehy.2015.08.013

Crosby, L., Davis, B., Joshi, S., Jardine, M., Paul, J., Neola, M., & Barnard, N. D. (2021).

Ketogenic diets and chronic disease: Weighing the benefits against the risks. *Frontiers in Nutrition, 8*(702802). https://doi.org/10.3389/fnut.2021.702802

Daisy Brand. (n.d.). *Southwestern omelette.* https://www.daisybrand.-com/recipes/southwestern-omelet-188/#tab-1574120172930-2-0

Daniela, G., Chiara, P., & Giuseppe, C. (2020). The possible role of ketogenic diet in fibromyalgia treatment. *Pharmacology Online, 3*(Special Issue), 122–126. https://phar-macologyonline.silae.it/files/specialissues/2020/vol3/PhOL_SI_2020_3_016_Guarino.pdf

Delish. (2016, June 29). *Beef & broccoli kebabs.* https://www.delish.com/cook-ing/recipes/a47945/beef-and-broccoli-kebabs-recipe/

Delish. (2020, August 26). *Keto pancakes.* https://www.delish.com/cooking/recipe-ideas/recipes/a58712/keto-pancakes-recipe/

Diabetes UK. (n.d.). *Ketones and diabetes.* https://www.diabetes.org.uk/guide-to-diabetes/managing-your-diabetes/ketones-and-diabetes

Diane. (n.d.). *Creamy garlic chicken recipe with broccoli (keto).* Eat Better Recipes. https://eatbetterrecipes.com/creamy-garlic-chicken/

Doubek, A. (2021, April 5). *Easy keto breakfast bowl with avocado.* Dancing through the Rain. https://dancingthroughtherain.com/easy-keto-breakfast-bowl/

Durrer, C., Lewis, N., Wan, Z., Ainslie, P., Jenkins, N., & Little, J. (2019). Short-term low-carbohydrate high-fat diet in healthy young males renders the endothelium susceptible to hyperglycemia-induced damage, an exploratory analysis. *Nutrients, 11*(3), 489. https://doi.org/10.3390/nu11030489

Eat This, Not That! (2019, October 3). *Keto frizzled eggs and sausage with sautéed greens recipe.* https://www.eatthis.com/keto-frizzled-eggs-sausage-recipe/

Eske, J. (2019, April 3). How does oxidative stress affect the body? *Medical News Today.* https://www.medicalnewstoday.com/articles/324863#:~:text=Oxidative%20stress%20-can%20damage%20cells

Garrard, C., & Alkon, C. (n.d.). *Will the keto diet help ease joint pain?* Everyday Health. https://www.everydayhealth.com/rheumatoid-arthritis/will-keto-diet-help-ease-joint-pain/

Gavin, J. (2021, January 1). What is the keto diet? *Jessica Gavin.* https://www.jessica-gavin.com/keto-diet-101/

Gladstone, L. (n.d.). Creamy pork chops with cauliflower mash. *Lena's Kitchen.* https://lenaskitchenblog.com/pork-chops-cauliflower-mash/#wprm-recipe-container-4253

Gore, M. (2020, February 27). *Keto beef stew.* Delish. https://www.delish.-com/cooking/recipe-ideas/a30996215/keto-beef-stew-recipe

Gorin, A. (2018, November 2). *The 11 biggest keto diet dangers you need to know about.* Everyday Health. https://www.everydayhealth.com/ketogenic-diet/diet/keto-diet-dangers-you-need-know/

Graff, S. (2019, April 11). A cardiologist's take on the keto diet. *Penn Medicine News Blog.* https://www.pennmedicine.org/news/news-blog/2019/april/a-cardiologists-take-on-the-keto-diet

Green, S. (2021, April 15). *Antioxidants: What are they and what are the top keto sources?* Ketogenic.com. https://ketogenic.com/antioxidants-what-are-they-and-what-are-the-top-keto-sources/

Harvard T.H. Chan School of Public Health. (2014a, May 15). *Saturated or not: Does type of fat matter?* The Nutrition Source. https://www.hsph.harvard.edu/nutrition-source/2014/05/15/saturated-or-not-does-type-of-fat-matter/

Harvard T.H. Chan School of Public Health. (2014b, June 9). *Types of fat.* The Nutrition Source. https://www.hsph.harvard.edu/nutritionsource/what-should-you-eat/fats-and-cholesterol/types-of-fat/#ref1

Harvard T.H. Chan School of Public Health. (2018, July 24). *Types of fat.* The Nutrition Source. https://www.hsph.harvard.edu/nutritionsource/what-should-you-eat/fats-and-cholesterol/types-of-fat/

Healthshots. (2019, December 31). *Thinking of embracing the keto diet in 2020? Read these 5 downsides first.* https://www.healthshots.com/healthy-eating/nutrition/be-aware-of-these-5-downsides-of-keto-diet-before-jumping-on-the-bandwagon/

Higuera, V. (2018, April 13). *Everything you need to know about keto breath.* Healthline. https://www.healthline.com/health/keto-breath

Holley, K. (2021, December 4). Old-fashioned keto meatloaf. *Peace, Love and Low Carb.* https://peaceloveandlowcarb.com/old-fashioned-keto-meatloaf/

Ketchum, C. (2020, April 12). *Salmon salad with avocado and spinach.* All Day I Dream About Food. https://alldayidreamaboutfood.com/keto-salmon-avocado-salad/

Ketogenic.com. (2021, August 19). *No appetite on keto? Here's why you aren't hungry.* https://ketogenic.com/no-appetite-on-keto-heres-why-you-arent-hungry/

Keto-Mojo. (2020, December 5). *11 significant health benefits of the ketogenic diet.* https://keto-mojo.com/article/top-11-health-benefits-of-keto/#

KetoVale. (2019, August 22). *Roasted lemon butter garlic shrimp and asparagus.* https://www.ketovale.com/roasted-lemon-butter-garlic-shrimp-and-asparagus/

Khan, N. (2021, January 27). *Cutting Carbs, Trying a Short Fast, and Other Ways to Get Into Ketosis.* Healthline. https://www.healthline.com/nutrition/7-tips-to-get-into-ketosis#2.-Include-coconut-oil-in-your-diet

Kingsland, J. (2020, September 8). Keto diet may reduce Alzheimer's risk by altering gut fungi. *Medical News Today.* https://www.medicalnewstoday.com/articles/keto-diet-may-reduce-alzheimers-risk-by-altering-gut-fungi

Krampf, M. (2016, June 4). Breakfast stuffed peppers (low carb, gluten-free). *Wholesome Yum.* https://www.wholesomeyum.com/recipes/cheesy-egg-stuffed-peppers/

Krampf, M. (2017, February 18). Keto paleo low carb granola cereal recipe - sugar-free. *Wholesome Yum.* https://www.wholesomeyum.com/recipes/low-carb-granola-cereal-paleo-gluten-free-sugar-free/

Krampf, M. (2019a, January 4). Low carb greek chicken meal prep bowls recipe. *Wholesome Yum.* https://www.wholesomeyum.com/low-carb-greek-chicken-meal-prep-bowls-recipe/#jumptorecipe

Krampf, M. (2019b, March 25). Coconut curry chicken: A keto low carb curry recipe. *Wholesome Yum.* https://www.wholesomeyum.com/keto-low-carb-curry-recipe/

Kubala, J. (2018, October 30). *What Is the Cyclical Ketogenic Diet? Everything You Need to Know.* Healthline. https://www.healthline.com/nutrition/cyclical-ketogenic-diet#basic-steps

Kubala, J. (2021, April 23). *9 potential intermittent side effects.* Healthline. https://www.healthline.com/nutrition/intermittent-fasting-side-effects

Kubala, J. (2022, January 4). *A keto diet meal plan and menu that can transform your body.* Healthline. https://www.healthline.com/nutrition/keto-diet-meal-plan-and-menu

Kwok, K. (2018, August 1). *Zucchini noodles with meatballs and tomato sauce (low carb/keto)*. Life Made Sweeter. https://lifemadesweeter.com/zucchini-noodles-with-meatballs/#wprm-recipe-container-34353

Kwok, K. (2019a, August 18). *Avocado egg boats*. Life Made Keto. https://lifemadeketo.com/avocado-egg-boats/

Kwok, K. (2019b, September 5). *Keto egg cups - 9 ways*. Life Made Keto. https://lifemadeketo.com/low-carb-breakfast-egg-muffins/

Lawler, M. (n.d.-a). *10 types of the keto diet to consider*. Everyday Health. https://www.everydayhealth.com/ketogenic-diet/diet/types-targeted-keto-high-protein-keto-keto-cycling-more/

Lawler, M. (n.d.-b). *The weird way the ketogenic diet affects your period*. Everyday Health. https://www.everydayhealth.com/ketogenic-diet/diet/your-period-how-keto-may-affect-your-cycle/

Lester, A., & Lester, L. (2020, February 5). *Steak and greens*. Cast Iron Keto. https://www.castironketo.net/blog/steak-and-greens/

Link, R. (2020, March 17). *Exercise on keto: Here's what to know*. Healthline. https://www.healthline.com/nutrition/working-out-on-keto#best-exercises-for-keto

Lite n' Easy. (2019, November 22). 7 benefits of meal planning. *Lite Bites*. https://www.lite-neasy.com.au/7-benefits-of-meal-planning/

Lumen Learning. (n.d.). *The citric acid (Krebs) cycle*. https://courses.lumenlearning.com/boundless-microbiology/chapter/the-citric-acid-krebs-cycle/#:~:text=The%20Krebs%20cycle%20is%20a

MacMillan, A. (2019, December 20). *7 dangers of going keto*. Health.com. https://www.health.com/weight-loss/keto-diet-side-effects

Mandal, A. (2019, February 27). *History of the ketogenic diet*. News Medical. https://www.news-medical.net/health/History-of-the-Ketogenic-Diet.aspx

Mawer, R. (2018, August 2). *10 Signs and Symptoms That You're in Ketosis*. Healthline. https://www.healthline.com/nutrition/10-signs-and-symptoms-of-ketosis#TOC_TITLE_HDR_10

Mawer, R. (2020, October 22). *The ketogenic diet: A detailed beginner's guide to keto*. Healthline. https://www.healthline.com/nutrition/ketogenic-diet-101#_noHeaderPrefixedContent

McDonald, S. (2020, October 4). *Keto cauliflower toast with avocado – Low carb breakfast recipe*. Tasteaholics. https://www.tasteaholics.com/recipes/breakfast-recipes/cauliflower-toast-with-avocado/

McSwiney, F. T., Doyle, L., Plews, D. J., & Zinn, C. (2019). Impact of ketogenic diet on athletes: Current insights. *Open Access Journal of Sports Medicine, 10*(2019), 171–183. https://doi.org/10.2147/OAJSM.S180409

The Meadowglade. (2019, December 26). *When eating disorders get rebranded*. https://themeadowglade.com/eating-disorders-rebranded/

Mensink, R. P., Zock, P. L., Kester, A. D. M., & Katan, M. B. (2003). Effects of dietary fatty acids and carbohydrates on the ratio of serum total to HDL cholesterol and on serum lipids and apolipoproteins: A meta-analysis of 60 controlled trials. *The American Journal of Clinical Nutrition, 77*(5), 1146–1155. https://doi.org/10.1093/ajcn/77.5.1146

MEpedia. (2021, July 26). *Ketogenic diet*. https://me-pedia.org/wiki/Ketogenic_diet

Migala, J. (n.d.). *Keto diet: A complete list of what to eat and avoid, plus a 7-day sample menu*.

Everyday Health. https://www.everydayhealth.com/diet-nutrition/ketogenic-diet/comprehensive-ketogenic-diet-food-list-follow/

Nazish, N. (2019, April 30). The essential guide to eating out on a keto diet. *Forbes.* https://www.forbes.com/sites/nomanazish/2019/04/30/the-essential-guide-to-eating-out-on-a-keto-diet/?sh=201d68961292

Nelson, S. (2021a, March 11). Portobello bun cheeseburgers. *Perfect Keto.* https://perfectke-to.com/portobello-bun-cheeseburgers/

Nelson, S. (2021b, April 30). Deliciously perfect keto creamed spinach. *Perfect Keto.* https://perfectketo.com/keto-creamed-spinach/

NHS. (2018, June 27). *What should my daily intake of calories be?* https://www.nhs.uk/common-health-questions/food-and-diet/what-should-my-daily-intake-of-calories-be/#:~:text=An%20ideal%20daily%20intake%20of

NHS. (2020, June 8). *Reference intakes explained.* https://www.nhs.uk/live-well/eat-well/what-are-reference-intakes-on-food-labels/

Nielsen, C. (2019a, July 23). Sugar-free chewy mocha chip cookies. *Perfect Keto.* https://perfectketo.com/mocha-chip-cookies/

Nielsen, C. (2019b, August 7). Delicious low-carb keto lasagna recipe. *Perfect Keto.* https://perfectketo.com/keto-lasagna/

Nielsen, C. (2021a, March 10). Weeknight Italian turkey casserole. *Perfect Keto.* https://perfectketo.com/italian-turkey-casserole/

Nielsen, C. (2021b, March 15). Zesty chili lime keto tuna salad recipe. *Perfect Keto.* https://perfectketo.com/chili-lime-keto-tuna-salad/

Oredola, T. (2020, July 24). Spicy cauliflower soup. *Low Carb Africa.* https://lowcar-bafrica.com/spicy-cauliflower-soup/

Pinto, A., Bonucci, A., Maggi, E., Corsi, M., & Businaro, R. (2018). Antioxidant and anti-inflammatory activity of ketogenic diet: New perspectives for neuroprotection in Alzheimer's disease. *Antioxidants, 7*(5), 63. https://doi.org/10.3390/antiox7050063

Popa, B. (n.d.). How to ace the keto diet with liposomal glutathione. *Core Med Science.* https://coremedscience.com/blogs/wellness/how-to-ace-the-keto-diet-with-liposomal-glutathione

QueenBea. (2018, December 8). *Rainbow trout with bok choy recipe.* Recipezazz.com. https://www.recipezazz.com/recipe/rainbow-trout-with-bok-choy-31036

Raman, R. (2020, February 20). *Building muscle on keto: A complete guide.* Healthline. https://www.healthline.com/nutrition/building-muscle-on-keto

Reisner, A. (2020, March 19). *37 healthy keto snack recipes for weight loss.* Eat This, Not That! https://www.eatthis.com/keto-snack-recipes-weight-loss/

Revers, J. (2021, July 20). *Avocado, egg & arugula salad with lemon balsamic vinaigrette.* A Cultivated Living. https://acultivatedliving.com/avocado-egg-arugula-salad-with-lemon-balsamic-vinaigrette/

Rico-Campà, A., Martínez-González, M. A., Alvarez-Alvarez, I., Mendonça, R. de D., de la Fuente-Arrillaga, C., Gómez-Donoso, C., & Bes-Rastrollo, M. (2019). Association between consumption of ultra-processed foods and all cause mortality: SUN prospective cohort study. *BMJ, 2019*(365), l1949. https://doi.org/10.1136/bmj.l1949

Rodal, R. (2019, November 15). Keto electrolytes: Tips and concerns. *Health Via Modern Nutrition.* https://hvmn.com/blogs/blog/ketosis-keto-electrolytes-tips-and-concerns

Rossano, J. (2019, September 16). Creamy coconut chia pudding. *NeuroticMommy*. https://neuroticmommy.com/2019/09/16/creamy-coconut-chia-pudding/

Rutherford, T. (n.d.). *One-pot keto zucchini alfredo*. Taste.com.au. https://www.taste.com.au/recipes/one-pot-keto-zucchini-lemon-alfredo-recipe/5gi89td4?r=healthy/x9a0fld8

Sadler, A. (2021, October 24). Quick and easy recipe: Keto egg muffins. *Perfect Keto*. https://perfectketo.com/keto-egg-muffins/

Scarfone, T. (2016, December 15). *Mocha chocolate chip cookies*. Joy Filled Eats. https://joyfilledeats.com/mocha-chocolate-chip-cookies/

Scarfone, T. (2020, November 12). *Keto chicken parmesan*. Joy Filled Eats. https://joyfilledeats.com/baked-chicken-parmesan/#recipe

Scher, B. (2021, July 30). *Carb cycling on a low-carb or keto diet: What you need to know*. Diet Doctor. https://www.dietdoctor.com/low-carb/carb-cycling

Sciarappa, P. (2021, July 24). *Keto chicken with mushrooms and asparagus in a creamy cheesy sauce*. Orsara Recipes. http://orsararecipes.net/keto-chicken-with-mushrooms-and-asparagus-in-a-creamy-cheesy-sauce

Seidelmann, S. B., Claggett, B., Cheng, S., Henglin, M., Shah, A., Steffen, L. M., Folsom, A. R., Rimm, E. B., Willett, W. C., & Solomon, S. D. (2018). Dietary carbohydrate intake and mortality: A prospective cohort study and meta-analysis. *The Lancet Public Health*, *3*(9), e419–e428. https://doi.org/10.1016/s2468-2667(18)30135-x

Shoemaker, S. (2020, August 11). *Top 13 keto-friendly drinks (besides water)*. Healthline. https://www.healthline.com/nutrition/keto-drinks-besides-water

Shoemaker, S. (2021, July 20). *What's the ideal ketosis level for weight loss?* Healthline. https://www.healthline.com/nutrition/ideal-ketosis-level-for-weight-loss#:~:text=Blood%20ketone%20levels%20while%20on

Shoemaker, S., & Spritzler, F. (2021, December 22). *20 Foods to eat on the keto diet*. Healthline. https://www.healthline.com/nutrition/ketogenic-diet-foods

Slajerova, M. (2021, July 18). *Creamy keto cinnamon smoothie*. KetoDiet App. https://ketodietapp.com/Blog/lchf/creamy-keto-cinnamon-smoothie

Slavin, J., & Carlson, J. (2014). Carbohydrates. *Advances in Nutrition, 5*(6), 760–761. https://doi.org/10.3945/an.114.006163

Slivinski, N. (n.d.). *Cancer and the keto diet*. WebMD. https://www.webmd.com/cancer/keto-diet-cancer-link

Sloam, J. (2016, May 9). *Cucumber salad with avocado and goats cheese*. Yummy Inspirations. https://yummyinspirations.net/2016/05/cucumber-salad/

Smith, C. (2021, June 14). *Marinated beef kabobs with broccoli (tender, flavorful)*. I Heart Umami®. https://iheartumami.com/beef-kabobs/

Spritzler, F. (2021, July 13). *How low carb and ketogenic diets boost brain health*. Healthline. https://www.healthline.com/nutrition/low-carb-ketogenic-diet-brain

Stark, E. (2016, April 27). *Recipe: Radish and turnip hash with fried eggs*. Kitchn. https://www.thekitchn.com/recipe-radish-and-turnip-hash-with-fried-eggs-230586

St-Onge, M.-P., Mayrsohn, B., O'Keeffe, M., Kissileff, H. R., Choudhury, A. R., & Laferrère, B. (2014). Impact of medium and long chain triglycerides consumption on appetite and food intake in overweight men. *European Journal of Clinical Nutrition, 68*, 1134–1140. https://doi.org/10.1038/ejcn.2014.145

Sullivan, K. (2021, November 25). *The ultimate guide to kitchen essentials*. Diet Doctor. https://www.dietdoctor.com/low-carb/keto/kitchen-essentials

Taylor, K. (2020, January 13). 6 keto diet-approved menu items major chains have rolled out across the US. *Insider*. https://www.businessinsider.com/keto-diet-approved-menu-items-at-chains-2019-8?IR=T

Thomas, C. (2020, February 7). *Keto stuffed jalapeños fat bomb*. Eat This, Not That!. https://www.eatthis.com/keto-fat-bomb-stuffed-jalapenos-recipe/

Upton, J. (2018, November 27). *The keto diet is super hard—These 3 variations are much easier to follow*. Health.com. https://www.health.com/weight-loss/keto-diet-types

Van De Walle, G. (2018, October 31). *The 7 best low-carb, keto-friendly protein powders*. Healthline. https://www.healthline.com/nutrition/low-carb-protein-powders#TOC_TITLE_HDR_9

Vibrance Med Spa. (2019, October 30). The keto diet and your skin. *Vibrance MedSpa Blog*. https://vibrancemedspa.com/the-keto-diet-and-your-skin/

Vicky. (2018, February 22). Low carb sushi rolls with smoked salmon and avocado. *Avocado Pesto*. https://avocadopesto.com/low-carb-sushi-rolls-salmon-avocado/

Volmer, M. (2020, October 19). *What's the best diet for chronic fatigue syndrome?* Flourish Clinic. https://fatiguetoflourish.com/whats-the-best-diet-for-chronic-fatigue-syndrome

Wallentin, J. (n.d.). *Sesame-crusted tuna steaks with wasabi mayo and bok choy*. Diet Doctor. https://www.dietdoctor.com/recipes/keto-sesame-crusted-tuna-steaks-with-wasabi-mayo-and-bok-choy

Winn, J. (2021, June 30). *Meatza (easy 10-minute prep recipe)*. The Real Simple Good Life. https://realsimplegood.com/meatza-low-carb-pizza-recipe/